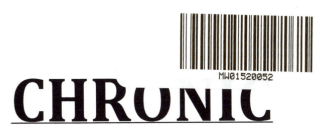

CHRONIC

THRIVING, NOT JUST
SURVIVING;
LIVING A LIFE WITH
CHRONIC ILLNESS

Nov 2016.

My copy!
K. E. Graham aka
Erica Worth

CONTENTS

An Introduction to my Own Personal Experience

After sharing what turned out to be a well received short article with readers of HypothyroidMom.com in 2014, I was encouraged to write a more comprehensive guide to how you can live a better and more fulfilled life, as you walk the path of Chronic Illness. I chose to use my own experiences as an example throughout this book, as it is far easier to explain things that way.

I would like to thank Dana Trentini for first giving me the opportunity to share some of my knowledge.

I was born in 1971 at Nocton Hall Hospital, Lincolnshire, England.

....Nocton Hall recently became famous as the setting for the movie Woman In Black 2!

I remember a very happy childhood, perhaps marred only by the fact that my biological father died three months before my birth, which I have always felt left a void.

At the age of six months, I was hastily returned to Nocton Hall Hospital having contracted Whooping Cough, which is also now known as Pertussis. I was chronically sick in the hospital ICU for six weeks, and unwell for at least eight months afterward.

I honestly don't think my immune system has ever recovered and that the pertussis may have been a catalyst for a lifetime of chronic illness. When I was four or five, I became aware that my maternal nana only had one leg. The other was amputated due to complications from diabetes. I saw this repeat situation in my later years, when my maternal aunt also endured an amputation for the same reason. It was in my mid twenties that I learned that my mom was also now diabetic. Through good choices and close monitoring, my mom is intact at the age of 71! She has shown signs of having autoimmune disease for many years. I see a cycle of some symptoms and some of the illnesses that mom went through, now repeating with me.

From the age of eight I remember feeling odd, and I really can't explain that feeling any differently. I would often get an upset stomach with instantaneous diarrhea, and debilitating headaches. I began having anxiety issues too. YES even at that young age.

My periods came when I was aged eleven, and almost immediately they were heavy, and they lasted for over a week at a time. I was skinny, restless, anxious, and I couldn't sleep. I had oily skin with acne, and greasy lank hair.

By age fourteen I had been prescribed sleeping medication, oral acne pills, and shots for migraine. My face was covered in acne, as was my back.

I was regularly visited in my home by a nurse counselor, who provided help in controlling depression and anxiety.

I contracted constant infections which were often bronchial in nature, and my sinuses were...and still are, akin to the 101 on a Los Angeles Monday morning!

On completion of school at the age of sixteen I attended college to become a hairdresser, after which I returned once more to Nocton Hall; this time to take employment as the in house hairdresser, while also working as a Nursing Assistant, at the Nursing Home there. I was in work one day and I remember starting to shake uncontrollably, I became incredibly anxious and my heart rate became incredibly fast. I was terrified by what was happening, because I had absolutely no idea what was causing this. The charge nurse had to drive me home that day, as I couldn't drive my car. I visited my family Dr. the next day and he prescribed beta blockers, with very little explanation as to what he thought my issue was, other than I was a little anxious. As far as I remember I didn't have a blood screen collected at this time.

If a blood screen was completed then my Dr. never relayed any of the results to me, and I stayed on

Beta Blockers for several years until I weaned myself off them.

I now know that this episode was very likely something serious possibly related to my thyroid, and that it could have been life threatening. I have experienced three similar episodes in the years since this first acknowledged one.

It was around this time, when I was aged twenty-two that the roller coaster of weight gain and loss started in earnest. I certainly never tried to lose or gain weight back then. I would likely have blamed working two jobs and taking an extra night shift here and there for the changes. That along with irregular sleep patterns, eating a student type diet, and partying a little too hard!

Down the road a little further at age twenty-eight, and very soon after the birth of my daughter, things just got worse...and worse. I began to experience chronic fatigue, depression and rapid weight gain, along with chronic pain in my hands, ankles, back, neck, wrists and shoulders.

I got heavier, sleepier, and more and more depressed. My hair fell out in handfuls. My Drs. blamed depression, and so the antidepressant Cipralex was the answer.

I always suspected a hormone imbalance, which made so much sense right after the birth of a child, but mine was not a medical opinion and so was largely ignored. I subsequently believed what the Drs. were saying.

In 2005, we immigrated from the UK, to Western Canada. Of course there is much stress involved in this process and I guess it must have finally taken it's toll.

Fast forward six more years years; and finally at age forty everything came to a head.

I was managing a clothing store at the time. I worked between fifty and sixty hours per week, in a store that had a two million dollar turnover every year. One day I went home from work feeling less than well.

I was halfway through my shift, which was not something that I ever considered doing. I was subsequently bedridden for over two weeks with influenza. The influenza was followed by a bout of what the Dr. called "standing pneumonia." My breathing became permanently labored and I began to cough chronically.

The cough was almost permanent for four years and though it is much improved now, I am still constantly breathless, and I still cough because of chronic allergic asthma and with overexertion. I take medication for this daily in the form of oral pills and multiple inhalers! I am also now living with with sleep apnea.

I am now forty-five years of age and though I do not feel great a lot of the time, I certainly believe that my Bio Identical Hormone Practitioner, who is also an OB/GYN, and my Respirologist (also an Internalist) have saved my life, merely by working with and listening to me.

They acknowledge my symptoms, trust my judgment, and accept my ability to relay how I feel.

Many Dr's won't work with patients in this manner, for whatever reason, and I'm a firm believer that it really can keep a person ill, and impede their ability to thrive when a Dr won't listen to what his patient is telling him.

I had lost 30lbs in the first year and a half since I was diagnosed with hypothyroidism and during that time I had been taking Natural Desiccated Thyroid (Erfa Thyroid) and other bio identical hormones. Now in peri menopause and with my weight fluctuating once more, I have been diagnosed as insulin resistant also. Victoza was added to my regimen and is slowing aiding the weight loss, but as I have modified my diet and added B1 vitamins I have been able to stop the Victoza, as my A1C numbers have dropped. I have made quite significant changes to my diet.

My Primary Care Provider, who is also a great listener, someone who really wants to help and has the ability to work with his patients has, over the past few years, randomly prescribed me pain medications, antibiotics and sleeping medication, but they tend to make me feel worse, so I try to stick to the bio-identical hormones, specialized breathing medications, vitamin supplements, and natural remedies.

I continue to undergo constant monitoring of my hormones, blood sugar and other illnesses and symptoms, including Hashimoto's Thyroiditis, Asthma, PCOS, Lupus, IBD and Cyclical Cushing's Syndrome.

Living with undiagnosed hypothyroidism and underlying illness until I was forty-two, culminating with my eventual insistence on full thyroid testing, has taken it's toll both physically and mentally. However throughout the years, I have always tried to do what I can when I am able, and I try to look good, and to stay positive about who I am. Of course, I'm a chronic illness patient so there are days when I don't even get dressed and my hairstyle is "ponytail." I absolutely feel that it is important to try to make an effort to stay positive and advocate for yourself. Without doubt you inevitably feel better when you look better and stay positive. There is definitely a psychological connect.

As an HNC/Associate Degree certified Esthetician/Beauty Therapist, and Massage Therapist, who has an extensive Anatomy and Physiology education, and five years experience working as a Nursing Assistant, I'm very lucky that I am educated enough to understand the human body and how we as humans function. This has helped me to know when things in my own body are different or changing. Education and life experience, often not great experiences, have helped me to be my own advocate, and I really hope that some of what I have learned and experienced will help you too.

My Personal Experiences and Symptoms

Over the course of a few weeks in early 2015, and shortly after my Endocrinologist began monitoring me for Cushing's Syndrome, I took the time to write down my symptoms. The ones that I could recall anyway.

There may still be a few missing. Some of these symptoms started over 30 years ago and some started very recently.

I offer this list as an aid that you may use, or as a guide for those that may be unsure if a symptom is real or not. This list can be used as a tool to compare your symptoms with others, or to perhaps explain to your Primary Care Provider, Endocrinologist etc, when they are telling you those symptoms are nothing, or that they are not related to one another. It is a long list, but descriptions have been kept brief and concise, as I know some of you are unable to concentrate for long periods.

Please feel free to edit, print, and use to help your own very important cause.

Long, and probably not complete list of chronic illness symptoms, that I have personally experienced, many of which I continue to suffer.

Head/Face:
Itchy, flaky, or scabs on scalp
Hair loss
Dry or brittle hair
Migraine type headache
Curly hair (from wavy or straight)
Grey hair
Swelling/water retention/Edema (Moon Face)
Acne (headless or boil type and other) In or behind the ears and on the chin
Oily Skin and enlarged pores
Red/high colored skin
Vitiligo/pigment changes
Facial hair growth (beard or mustache)
Excessive lanugo hair on cheeks
Facial tic on nose
Sinus/Ear/Throat infections

Loss of smell
Swollen (crimped) tongue

Eyes:
Vision disturbance, changing level of vision
Light intolerance
Puffy skin around eyes, definition of eye changes
Tic
Floaters
Dryness
Excessive watering

Ears:
Tinnitus (buzzing, hissing, high pitch noise)
Hearing disturbance or loss (fuzzy)
Infections; ear, nose and throat

Neck Shoulders Arms Hands Upper torso:
Hypothyroidism; including swelling and goiters
Infections; chest
Skin tags
Buffalo hump
Weak, grating or painful shoulders
Supraclavicular (fat pads at base of neck and shoulders) pads
Excessive sweating
Increase in moles or freckles (on hands also)

Acne
Underarm stretch marks
Breast growth with stretch marks
Brittle/peeling fingernails nails

Torso:
Fat increase on belly/back
Stretch marks
Distended belly
Pain in kidney area
Low back pain
Hair on belly/abdomen

Digestive:
Heartburn
Bloating
Constipation
Diarrhea
Farting/Gas
Metal taste in mouth
Thirst
Hunger
Frequent urination
Glucose intolerance
Awfully painful radiating pain through chest and upper back, comes in waves. Lasts anywhere from 1-3 hours

Menstrual:
Periods lasting 14+ days
Heavy bleeding (super tampons falling out after 1/2 an hour)
Blinding debilitating migraine headaches
Cravings for salt and sugar
Chronic fatigue
Memory and thought disturbance
Increased acne with oily skin and hair
Excessive sweating
Diarrhea
Increased palpitations
Mood swings
Perimenopause
Menopause

Incidental and affecting the entire body:
Chronic fatigue
Breathlessness with chronic cough
Breathless with little or no effort
Dizziness
Heart palpitations
Weakness in limbs/hands/feet//back/shoulders
Shooting pains
Loss of grip
Vertigo
Insomnia and Sleep Apnea
Total exhaustion
Depression
Anxiety
Aphasia; inability to converse. Words jumbled, not able to find descriptive words. Poor memory and confusion.
Chronic bone and/or muscle pain
Cramping
Pins and needles
Unexplained bruises
Dry skin

Noise intolerance
Libido changes
Hives

Hips, Legs and Feet:
Plantar warts
Dry cracked skin
Plantar fasciitis
Weak/painful/burning feet ankles
Shooting pains generally in knees and ankles
Edema
Restless Leg Syndrome (RLS)
Cracking/grating hips with pain
Knee cracking/pain
Purpura
Hirsute thighs

To add a little more insight into my treatment, I decided to include this list of medical tests (and results) that I underwent between August 2011 and April 2015

C-Reactive protein **Double what is considered normal**(Inflammation)
Antistreptolysin count **Double what is considered normal** (infection)
A1C Insulin **Double what is considered to be normal** (Insulin resistance)
Anti TPO **HIGH** (Hashimoto's Thyroiditis)
Low B12
Low Vitamin D
Low morning Cortisol (from blood test)

24 hour urine test:
Creatinine **Low**
DHEA's **Low**
Cortisol 24 Hr **(Above range by 25%)**

24 Hr Cortisone **(High end of range)** (Cushing's Disease)

Metabolized Cortisol **(Above Range by 60%)**
Tetrahdrocortisols **(all above range by 50%)**
ACTH **Low**

The above can also all be linked to Lupus, yet no-one would give me a Lupus diagnosis for three years.

CT scan Oct 2011
Altered liver enzymes or mildly hyperechoic (presumably fatty) (Hashimoto's Thyroiditis)
Small kidney cysts upper pole of left kidney 9mm and 11 mm

CT July 2012
Incidental (left) liver **cysts**
16 mm cyst on anterior aspect of pancreas (nonspecific, but likely incidental cyst) possibly due to previous pancreatitis **(Lupus)**
Several small renal cysts

CT Aug 2012
Cardiopericardial silhouette mildly enlarged (CT ratio 0.56) likely secondary to cardiomegaly **(Lupus)**
13 mm Splenule adjacent to splenic hilum
Degenerative changes in lower thoracic spine

As I previously stated; in August 2011 I suddenly became very (chronically) sick.

For a full twelve months following this my (then) Dr. relayed none of these imaging findings, or test results to me.

Only when I was required to collect this information for my insurance provider in early 2014, and three years after the original CT and blood tests, was I made aware of any of these issues.

So to reiterate; I only became aware of these test results when I personally had to collect paperwork for my insurance provider.

Time and again I was fobbed off and diagnosed with obesity, depression and fibromyalgia. Even though all of this information was in my file. Never once was further investigation done.

Eventually I decided to pay $400 of my own money to see a Dr privately. Five weeks prior to our appointment I was required to have fifteen vials worth of blood testing, along with urine samples. This very blood work tested my hormones and other levels, and found thyroid, hormone, adrenal, inflammation, and antibody abnormalities. All of which required medication that was not an anti depressant, sleeping pill, or a pain medication.

I was eventually urged to do further adrenal testing, which showed yet further illness.

Only because I continued to push for answers are we now at a place with diagnosis and the correct treatment.
You must also push too.

Self advocation is so very necessary.

It can be time consuming, frustrating, upsetting and at times a little costly on the pocket book, but it is very necessary, and it is so very worth the effort and cost.
In 2015 my current PCP apologized for taking so long to find me a diagnosis, told me he was sorry that he hadn't fully believed what I was telling him at times, and then agreed that I was right in both my suspicions, and in my insistence to test..and keep testing.

He then attempted to prescribe me opiates so that I could exercise pain free..... Oh well, you can't win 'em all.

UPDATE. It turns out I'm blessed with Hashimoto's Thyroiditis, Cyclical Cushing's Syndrome, Polycystic Ovary Syndrome, Lupus, Chronic Allergic Asthma, I'm Peri menopausal and I have a topping of Insulin Resistance...
I'm also shorter by half inch

It really shouldn't be this hard.

What Is a Chronic Illness?

When you first become ill, you may not realize that you have a chronic illness. You may not even consider it for quite a long period of time. *

As you remain sick for a longer period of time, you will begin to undergo medical testing of all manner, perhaps medicine will be prescribed to you, and a care plan may be discussed between you and your Dr. or medical team. You will possibly soon come to suspect that what you are living with is indeed a chronic illness.

Your Dr. may never disclose this information to you in such words. No-one has ever said to me "you have a chronic illness or disease," despite the fact that I do in fact have several illnesses that are considered to be chronic. I received a random phone call in December of 2014 asking me to visit a Nurse Practitioner at my Drs. office, so we could discuss a chronic care plan.

Unfortunately at that time the wrong "chronic" thing was addressed, we were already three years into my illnesses changing my life in so many ways, and it still took a further six months to get a referral to an Endocrinologist, someone I would have benefited from meeting with at least 20 years ago!

Once your condition is acknowledged, either by the Dr. giving you the name of an illness that is considered chronic, confirming that what you have is indeed considered a chronic disease, or through your own research, realization and experiences, you need to know the following;

A chronic disease or illness is a something that is usually life changing, constant, and generally permanent; though often with varying levels of severity, remissions, and flares. It may become impossible for you to plan your life as you are used to doing, and you may find that you may have to live day to day for the near future, possibly for the rest of time. You may have to stop working. You might have to discontinue some of your hobbies. You might well have to stop doing your own housework and chores. Well, that last one may not be so tough, huh?

Many of these things can be terrifying to even consider. I would urge you to hang in there. It really is just a matter of patience, education, understanding, tolerance and adjustment for the most part.

Living with a chronic illness or disease can be a constant and hard battle, a long tough road. However, you can live with and tolerate most of what a chronic illness throws at you.

You can survive and many of you will thrive, and you can avoid the chaos and stress that initially occurs with a new situation or diagnosis, if you are patient, organized, and dedicated to your cause. Chronic disease will almost inevitably change you as a person; both physically and mentally. You will undoubtedly be restricted in what you can achieve. Your perspective on almost everything will change. At your lowest points you may feel pain, frustration, anger, sadness, and even depression. Those around you may not be able to easily understand or cope with the difficulties and changes that occur. If those people become too negative, and cause you additional stresses on a regular basis, you may have to make the decision to let them go.

This will prove to be upsetting and challenging in itself, but in releasing negative energy from your life, you will see the benefit almost immediately. I have lost friends and family because I refuse to have them negatively affecting my life. I don't have the tolerance for them, and I certainly don't have the time for games, drama and ignorance and you should not tolerate these behaviours either.

It is very important to remember that you do not have to do things to please anyone else. Adjust to your differing lifestyle slowly, and tailor it to suit your physical and mental abilities. Rest when you are tired. Try to stay stimulated when you can. Find a lifestyle that is within your means and do at least one thing that you enjoy on a daily basis.

Listen to music, read poetry, take photographs, paint, write a letter, cook, go for a short walk...you get the idea. Time out for yourself is very important when dealing with a chronic illness. You can, indeed you will have good, even great days. Not every day will be good, but some of them will be, and every effort you put into doing something will be so worth your time and energy. You will be proud of yourself. Heck, I sat and wrote a book. I hadn't written in close to this capacity since I revisited college to study for my HNC in 2002! OK, so it was a year long process, but I still did it.

No one person will have the exact symptoms as another, and you may at times require some assistance, you may not. Getting help is not something to be embarrassed about. Take any help that you feel you need. Ask for help if you feel you should. Consider always when embarking on something that may cause you pain or discomfort "Is it necessary?" "Can I delegate?" "Can it wait for a few days?" If the answer is "no, no, and yes," you are free to take a mineral bath, or read a book.

If it can't wait, split the task down, and do it at your own pace.

If your health care team suggests a medication, or regimen and you agree with them, go ahead and try it. If you don't agree, and you are absolutely not obliged to, you should always feel free to discuss things further. Request an alternative. If you do try something and it is not working for you, revisit your Dr. when you are able, to discuss an alternative. There are always options. Something that may have worked for you for years could be less successful as your illness progresses, or when your symptoms change. Addressing any change in a situation quickly and decisively, is always the best option. Don't ever rest on your laurels. Advocate for yourself, and if you can't, have someone close to you negotiate on your behalf.

You need to be able to concentrate on living a life that is fulfilling and manageable.

Here is a less than comprehensive list of some diseases that are considered chronic. You may have more than one. That is not considered unusual, but it can complicate things a little more.

- Addison's disease
- ALS
- Asthma
- Arthritis
- Bipolar disorder
- Bronchiectasis
- Cancer
- Cardiac failure
- Cardiomyopathy
- Chronic obstructive pulmonary disease
- Chronic kidney disease
- Coronary artery disease
- Crohn's disease
- Cushing's disease
- Depression
- Diabetes Insipidus
- Diabetes mellitus (type 1 and type 2)
- Dysrhythmia (irregular heartbeat)
- Epilepsy
- Eczema
- Fibromyalgia
- Glaucoma

- Haemophilia
- HIV
- Hyperlipidaemia (high cholesterol)
- Hypertension (high blood pressure)
- Hyperthyroidism (overactive thyroid)
- Hypothyroidism (inactive thyroid gland)
- Metabolic Syndrome
- Multiple Sclerosis
- Parkinson's disease
- Polycystic Ovary Syndrome
- Psoriasis
- Rheumatoid arthritis
- Schizophrenia
- Systemic lupus erythematosus
- Ulcerative colitis

* In Western medical fields, an illness is considered chronic after a period of three months.

Are You Sick?

Are you sick? Do you know, or do you care for someone who is sick?
If the answer is yes, then you, or the person you know, would almost definitely benefit from reading this book.

As you will see when you read on, the discovery of my chronic illness emerged over a period of thirty plus years. I had odd symptoms here and there, which although awful, seemed to be unconnected to one another.
In reading this book you will learn to understand how seemingly random infections, rashes, mobility issues, etc. may be connected. You will also learn how to at least try to piece together that puzzle of confusion.
My aim is to not burden you with statistics or jargon. I know how difficult it can be to digest

information and just simply navigate life when you are ill.

My aim is more to awaken in you a realization of the implications of your illness, and to guide you through some of the steps of living and dealing with long term or chronic illness, that you may find helpful.

In the progression of a chronic illness at whatever age, you may experience any one, some, or all the following.

You may have more symptoms that you are not really aware of, or symptoms that the Dr. attributes to aging, or a natural progression. Even if you are only aged twenty or thirty, your Dr. is probably fobbing you off when he says that you illness is a natural sign or symptom of ageing...Look around you, not everyone at age forty needs to take a nap every day. Besides, you have probably been experiencing debilitating fatigue for ten or more years now, right?
I hope that in reading this you will learn to reasonably assess and process all and any information that you, those close to you, and your medical, with the aid of recommended internet

tools, collect and are offered, and you can use that information to best help your individual situation. REMEMBER this; No two people with Multiple Sclerosis have identical symptoms or prognosis.

One person with Chronic Plaque Psoriasis may have a covered torso, another may be experiencing facial coverage. Osteoporosis may prevent one person from walking, while another is feeling pain only in their hands and knees.

The same applies to EVERY single illness and every single person on earth. Not one of us is a textbook case.

We, along with our very individual (however similar they may appear) diseases, need personalized and tailored care, perhaps what is more important is that we MUST learn to advocate for that care.

ALWAYS be very aware that normal is a setting on the tumble dryer, and should rarely be considered for discussion when appearing on a blood panel.

If normal is a range from 2-10, surely we want to be at the optimal point on that range? I know I do. Weight, height, climate and diet, often along with many other factors, will mean that your normal is not even similar to someone else's. Illness is not cut and dried, it is rarely ever simple and you must also feel well in order to be considered "normal", despite what a blood test says.

Here are a few of the more serious symptoms of chronic illness that you should seek immediate help for, although it is very likely that by the time these symptoms are noticed, you will probably already be quite sick.

Fatigue is top of my list, because by the time we become fatigued, we have likely been experiencing several, or many other symptoms, and tolerating them for a good period of time.
If you wake in the morning and feel tired; something is not right. No ifs, ands and buts.
If you need a nap..two naps, or more during the day, you need to see a Dr. right away.

Insomnia and sleep disturbances are often symptoms of chronic or prolonged illness. Insomnia may be a symptom of disease, or it could be caused by medication you already use. Either way it is disruptive and annoying at the very least. Insomnia can be very serious and it should always be investigated.

Pain is on this list because it can be can be so entirely life changing and can be linked to almost

every chronic illness out there. I strongly believe that pain is not generally a stand alone disease, yet a symptom of what are usually more well understood, yet in many individual cases are likely under investigated, or ignored illnesses. ANY pain, however random or slight is your body telling you that something is not okay.
Always have pain investigated.

Weight gain or loss, sudden, or over a period of time. If your routine, diet and lifestyle have not changed, but your weight has, seek the advice of a Dr. soon. Often you will notice a digestive disturbance or perhaps a change in the desire to consume food.

Visual changes, more often degraded vision, can be a sign that there is an underlying illness.

 Headaches which become frequent, or are prolonged are always a cause for concern.

Depression or long episodes of unhappiness. It is not normal for someone to be depressed.
If your general outlook is "blah," you should seek advice, at the very least.
Your medical team should always investigate any signs of depression.

Memory loss, poor concentration, inability to communicate as effectively as you previously could. I had an excellent memory...and then I didn't. I was thirty-eight when this became more noticeable, to myself at least. Now my medications are what I would consider close to optimal, my memory, concentration, and communication, are far greater again.

Mobility changes. Of course if you are less mobile you likely have other symptoms. Loss of mobility should be investigated immediately.

Motor skills that have worsened or become poor. If you lose the ability to fasten buttons or hold a knife and fork, even for a day here or there, you really need to visit a Dr. and have a thorough physical and perhaps further testing.

Skin lesions, hives or color variants, generally indicate a change in tolerance, immunity and severity of disease. This includes new or worsening allergies.

REMEMBER that just because a symptom is mild, you only experience it every few months, or you are only recently experiencing one or more symptoms, it is very possible that you may already be seriously ill. Any changes, especially ones that cause a

disruption to your ability to live a normal life,
warrant an immediate and thorough investigation.

Are You a Specialist?

As I sat at my desk writing this book, I absolutely
acknowledged that I am not medically qualified to
prescribe you a pill, or refer you to a specialist.

But then I asked myself this question;
What makes a someone a specialist?

I have a strong desire to help you and those around
you, and just like those that I have called upon to

help me, I know a lot about chronic illness. Perhaps more than I am comfortable with knowing at times. Strangers have often, without requesting payment and not questioning the amount of time that I had taken, or what I was asking of them, just wanted to help me because they have lived in my situation, and they saw in me, what they themselves are. These advocates are experienced and they are educated, because they have lived through a chronic real life experience.

Are these advocates real life Specialists? I believe so. I am educated in Anatomy and Physiology as part of an HNC/Associate Degree in Esthetics/Beauty Therapy and massage. I understand the human body and its systems, and I know how those systems function separately, and in partnership with each other. I have a certificate that states it, but that doesn't make me a Dr.

Often, a Dr has a certificate, but no real life experience and very little knowledge or real understanding, of what you are trying to relay to him.

How many of the Drs. that we visit live 24/7 live with the illness or condition that they treat? Very few is the answer.

When they learn about these conditions in school, is what they see in a hospital or clinic setting the complete illness? Likely it is a very minute snippet of that illness. A Snapchat moment of illness if you will. A Dr. would have to spend at least six months in my home to see the full cycles and consequences of my illness.

What Drs. are likely to see is;

Mrs Adams 42; presenting with chronic pain, poor memory and weight gain.

Mr Brooks 28; here with a chronic cough, labored breathing, body wide skin lesions and weight loss.

Susan Keene 35; has had issues with heavy menstruation for over twenty years, is now in chronic pain, has hair loss, and is experiencing high C reactive protein levels.

How long is an average Dr. visit? Maybe 15 minutes maximum...

In those fifteen minutes will the Dr. listen to the patient, or merely refer to a few blood panels and dismiss the very apparent physical symptoms as; obviously caused by an eating issue, lack of exercise, depression or ageing.

I'm sure this paints a pretty clear picture. Most of us living with a chronic condition (or two, or three) could, and probably should be considered experts in that condition. Yet a person who has never lived it, gets to make all of the decisions and choices for us, regarding medications and treatments.

This book is not and cannot be used as medical advice.
It is written purely from my experiences and the experiences of others that I have spoken with.

I'd like for you to use this book to gain a fresh perspective on your situation and condition. To learn to adapt and reevaluate, to banish negative experiences and ideals, and to perhaps guide you to advocate for yourself more. I want you to learn to look at the positive and for you to revel in even the tiniest improvement or change for the better.

You must become Specialist in the condition, disease or illness you live with, in order that you can thrive, and not to just survive.
Take the time and learn to interpret your blood panels, body imaging, and lab work.
Encourage your Dr. to explain these results to you. This is one of the most necessary things that you can do as a self advocate. When you know what these

test results mean for yourself, you can push to get better, improved, or alternative treatment.

I'd like to think I can provide at least one light bulb moment on your journey through what, however awful it is at any given time, can also be an educational and enlightening experience.

This is THE guide for realization, education and self preservation while living life CHRONIC.

DON'T just SURVIVE… YOU deserve to THRIVE.

Testimonials By People Living With a Chronic Illness

I know many other people who unfortunately tread the same path as me every day.

With that in mind, I made a polite request to some friends who live with chronic diseases and illnesses, to ask them if they would be able to tell me what

they found most debilitating about their illness, and how it made them feel on the whole..
Here are the very candid answers of those who replied.

Lucy Caine is a Legal Assistant who lives in England, and she said this; "I suffer from a chronic condition called Benign Paroxysmal Positional Vertigo, or BPPV, which is a balance disorder. This means that I often suffer from a spinning sensation which upsets my vision and motion, causing sickness and brain fog. Not life threatening, just debilitating. To describe what I miss the most is; The ability to plan ahead. I often have to cancel plans, not because want to do it, just because I feel too shit."

Jackie Scott has Hashimoto's Thyroiditis. Jackie is a Hairstylist from England; "I miss just being able to do things without having to think about the fatigue and pain that will come for days after." Is what Jackie shared. Simple and to the point, but Jackie's simple explanation is all some of us will need to make the connection.

Mark Power lives in Alberta, Canada, and he was diagnosed with Multiple Sclerosis, which is also known as MS, over five years ago. Here is what Mark said; "I'm not the writing person by any means, but I can say a lot about being in a Supervisory Position in the Oil Field. I went days off from my job in September 2010 and haven't worked a day since, because while I was home I was diagnosed with Multiple Sclerosis.

At the time it didn't seem sudden because I only thought I was going to be off for a few weeks until they figured out a treatment for me, but that was over five years ago and in the first six months of that, I had four massive attacks that left me disabled for life.

Pretty much put me in a wheelchair full time. I became housebound. I decided to put my foot down and fight this monster, so I flew to Newport Beach California and got my Chronic Cerebrospinal Venous Insufficiency (CCSVI) treatment done, not once, but twice in a little over a month.

That gave me the energy to attend physiotherapy two-three times a week. The rest is history, I go fishing and I'm as active as I can be. I'm living life to the fullest. Do I miss work some days? YES... other days no. The biggest thing bothering me these days, is having to have people attend to me at times and forever asking for help with common everyday things."

Carla Cumiskey used to be a dog groomer, and is now a full time Mom. Carla lives in England and was diagnosed with Myalgic Encephalopathy or ME several years ago. More recently came a diagnosis of bipolar type 2. She had this to say;

"For me, the pains, aches and fatigue are bad, but they pale in comparison to the loss of memories. Memories of my son growing up, memories of happy times, memories of a life I have lived. It may not be a 'normal' life as others can live, periods of not working and doing activities I most enjoy, but what I have done and the times I have enjoyed (which are many) are often forgotten, or dumbed by blank spaces or black clouds of depression, haunted you could say by all the bad things. Don't get me wrong, living a normal life would be wonderful, but I myself am far from normal and I'm ok with that."

VJ is an Holistic Professional from the Pacific North West of the United States, and was only very recently diagnosed with Hypothyroidism, which subsequently required that she have a partial thyroidectomy. This is her story;

"I've been struggling with fatigue and extreme body pain, mostly in my joints, but also upper shoulders and back, the cold sensations in my body are so deep I can't ever get warm, I've had weight gain when I'm barely eating, and numbness in hands and feet for years. All my blood work always came back as 'normal'. Eventually I developed a large cyst on the left side of my thyroid that sat near my windpipe, and caused severe pain and discomfort. Finally doctors are addressing the thyroid issue and the years of physical challenges.

What's been the hardest for me is losing my ability to be as active as I used to be. I used to love to go on long hikes, and ride my bike to go on my adventures. Now it's an achievement to go for a nice walk. What's hard is feeling physically older than I am and feeling limited by the pain in my body. Also, learning to offer myself love and acceptance with a very different body and appearance than I am used to. The weight gain and pain has changed my 'youthful' appearance, and makes it hard to like what I see when I look in a mirror.

I have worked in the holistic healthcare field for years and have helped many people release physical issues connected to unresolved emotional patterns, and so Initially I felt like I had failed myself, that I shouldn't have been in this position of illness. But I've made peace with that and am moving forward with a blend of Allopathic medicine, as well as alternative healing to reclaim my health.

I'm looking forward to increased energy and vitality, and being able to move with ease and strength and feeling good in my body!"

Shellie Blow is from England. Shellie is an extremely talented artist and dressmaker, who now lives with Fibromyalgia or FMS, and Fuch's Endothelial Dystrophy or FED. Shellie tells it as it is: "I first realised something 'wasn't quite right' in December 2012. I was decorating my daughter's bedroom, wallpapering and painting, something I loved to do and could do with ease. Only it wasn't easy. In fact it was bloody painful. My arms, shoulders and back were on fire. I thought maybe I was just out of shape, and the extra effort on my muscles was the reason for the pain. But it didn't go away. The bedroom didn't get finished. I got diagnosed with Fibromyalgia.

Since then there have been an awful lot of things which haven't got finished, but even more which haven't even got started.

Fibromyalgia has taken away so many thing which I used to take for granted, it has also given me some things which I really would prefer not to have.

I know when I am being defeatist, I'm not so far down the spiral that I can't see myself, and I am the first to admit to the odd bout of self-pity. It's impossible to stay upbeat when you can't make firm plans with friends and family because you don't know if you'll be physically able to even get out of bed, let alone get showered and dressed to go out for dinner.

But It's not all bad. I have learned that some things just aren't worth bothering about. Where I used to save the good stuff for 'best', I just use it, because now might be 'best' and I'd rather use it all up than be left wishing.

I am told to pace myself, don't do too much, take rest, take care of myself.

I also just got diagnosed with Fuch's Endothelial Dystrophy. FED is a degenerative disease of the cornea. It affects your sight. Eventually my vision may be so bad that I will need a cornea transplant. Pacing myself and not doing too much now seems impossible. How can I take my time? I need to do it now, while I can still see to do it.

So I guess I'll just carry on doing too much. The bad days will be worse than they might have been, but the good days will be infinitely better than they would have been."

Kimberley Core, who is from Ontario, Canada, shared her story and it just shows that whether we have disease, or our affliction is borne through accident, we all face the same challenges. Here is Kimberley's story; "After an injury I needed emergency surgery to remove herniated disc tissue that was compressing my spinal cord, and making it so that I couldn't feel my legs or even walk. The surgery was largely a success, and I've been back to work several years, but I'll never be 100% again. I work IT in the healthcare industry as a programmer/support analyst. For me one of the hardest things is that visibly you can't see that anything is wrong, so it's easy for others to forget. My colleagues often book long meetings where it's disruptive to have to stand up or shift, or they book meetings an hour away, when I can't drive that far. It's like a constant reminder of the things I can't do, and having to say it feels uncomfortable, like I'm looking for sympathy. It's sometimes embarrassing.

I put all of my energy into working, so when I'm home there's nothing left. I'm too sore to do anything with the family, and I can't always keep up with what needs to be done around the house, which means no visitors because I don't want anyone to see a mess!"

All of these stories are told by people who were forty years of age or younger, when they first experienced symptoms, some of whom went through years of visiting a Dr. yet were ignored, or told that they were normal.
Each one of these people shows that perseverance and self advocation does indeed lead to a path of thriving, and not merely surviving.
All are self advocates, but all still face a daily battle.

Adapting Your Life; Changing Your Lifestyle

If you have always been an active person, changing
your lifestyle to include less activity and less
physical or mental exertion, can be very traumatic,
and may take years of adjustment. In addition, any
changes that are made are likely to be permanent.
You must be willing to educate yourself, and there is
a chapter in this book on how to do exactly that.
Then you need to help educate your friends and
family. Finally you will need to make the necessary
adjustments required in your specific case, this

should enable you to live happily and healthily with any restrictions you may have.

What you absolutely MUST AWAYS to do is focus on you. Focus on what makes YOU happy, and how best YOU can handle any situation you find yourself in.

Learn to never be apologetic or embarrassed about your physical appearance, any lack of vitality, or the way you feel. Ensure right from the onset of learning to live with your illness, that those around you never berate or belittle you, and certainly never tolerate this behaviour from strangers who do not know you, or your situation.

This can be immensely frustrating if you have a disabled or handicapped parking badge, but require no sticks, walking aids or a wheelchair. Some people are quick to judge, they cannot see the pain and fatigue, or the sheer effort that it takes you to walk into, and around the store.

You may get looks, and sideways glances. If this happens, look these folk dead in they eye. Mostly they will be shocked and move along. If however, someone approaches you and asks why you are parked in a space that is marked for a disabled person, feel free to set them straight. Be polite and to the point. You don't have to justify or explain your illness to anyone, least of all a judgemental stranger.

You will almost certainly find yourself visiting your Drs. more frequently as a result of your illness. Try and schedule your appointments for times that are suitable for you and not at a time that is convenient for the Dr. YOU are the important person here. The Dr. is working for you.

You may have a good amount of energy one day, but not the next three.
You might find that you need some help with chores, such as laundry, cleaning and grocery shopping.
Maybe it will help to establish a daily routine, there are times that you will have to adapt daily.
All of these adjustments may take weeks, months, or even years, for you to figure out and fine tune.
The trick is not to let frustration get the better of you. Adjust, tweak, and readjust.
Take the time you need. This is your health and your life, it's not a race. You will absolutely be the winner in every scenario.

Many people find that as part of a chronic illness, their social life inevitably becomes an antisocial life. Friends...REAL friends, will agree to learn about your illness and they will adapt to your needs and requirements. Some will become a great help and will even advocate for you. Other people will fall by the wayside...and you must let them go. Negative and dramatic people are not a healthy addition to any chronic illness, they are restrictive and they will hamper your well being, and your desire to thrive. If you are feeding the negativity of others, you are wasting the vital energy that you need to progress, and you cannot let that happen if you want to lead a fulfilled and happy existence.

There really is no need for further discussion of this right now.

If you were a person who was used to visiting a bar every weekend, or maybe you loved volunteering with the local charity, you may now find that you are unable to do that any more and if you are still able, it may be on a much less frequent basis.

Any of these adjustments and changes can be demoralizing and cause anger and frustration, they may lead to depression.

Quickly ask your Dr. to refer you to a councillor if are ever feeling low or depressed, and you think that some discussion may help you to figure out what is the best course of action for you. Often, just talking something over can initially help you to straighten out in your mind what is causing these feelings of sadness. Maybe just by reading this book you will better understand that being chronically ill is not your fault, and that you cannot always control the outcome when dealing with something as complex as your health. I have referred myself to a councillor on more than one occasion and she has been really helpful. Of course I have still had to work on my own feelings and how best to live with my situation, but having a guide is generally a good thing.

If you were an outdoor type person before you became ill, perhaps you were into horse riding, cycling or even kayaking, and you cannot do these things right now, you must learn to compromise but not to ostracize yourself. Go to those events and be a spectator, help to set up the refreshment tables, or volunteer at the local stable when you have a good day. You can easily stay involved, just on a lesser scale and at your leisure.

Being able to partake in just the simplest of hobbies such as knitting and writing, can become difficult with a chronic illness. Arthritis is just one of the debilitating diseases that will absolutely hamper your motor skills. Other illnesses will bring pain and fatigue, along with brain fog, or memory issues, that can make other hobbies hard to be involved in. You will inevitably feel low at one time or another. It is a natural progression with such an immense reconstruction of your life.

If you can learn not to schedule the the fun things, rather learn to do them when you have the urge or ability it will be much easier for you. Make a small and reasonable list of the things you want to produce or work through, but don't restrict them with a timeline. Slow and steady really does win this race.

Restricting the fun things in life will only lead to further frustrations that you really don't need. You need to be able to still do things on a whim if at all possible.
If you are one of those people that is awake late at night or early into the morning, and you feel that you can, you should absolutely use that time to get creative. You'd be likely sitting around feeling lost, or watching CNN on a loop as an alternative.

Writing down ideas for things you would like to acheive can be done at any time, so always keep a notebook, laptop, or your cell phone beside you. Noting things down right away will not only help you to remember those ideas, but it also will free up your brain and help you to focus on the now.

Do you have a yard? You can easily set it up so that birds and critters will visit. I have a real menagerie of birds, ranging from Woodpeckers and Jays, to Finches and Crows. I often see small animals just because I put out a few bird feeders and a birdbath. I let the grass get a little longer in certain spots to encourage rabbits and voles.
Recently a new Momma squirrel has been visiting.

Of course, my yard cannot be perfect anyway, I suffer far too frequently from pain and fatigue. I don't have the energy to manicure it perfectly, but it is beautiful. It is a quite a large space and to fill in the gaps, my husband has planted many bushes, trees and wildflowers.

It's not symmetrical and will never win best kept, but it now serves a great purpose.

Early in my illness I found that going to the hairdressers was a grind. I have longer hair and I used to get highlights or a color every 3 months. I quickly found that I could not sit in the chair for the three hour period that it took to make me look different. I stopped visiting my stylist for almost three years and grew out the color.

As a former hairdresser, I was knowledgeable enough to be able to cut and style my own hair. Three years later I discovered that I have the most gorgeous natural colored hair. I still keep it fairly long, but now visit my stylist every three months or so. We do change the style here and there, but being color free keeps my appointment time to an acceptable forty minutes.

I know that in writing this book I absolutely focus most on the things I would personally do.

I'd like to make a brief apology because of that, but I want to also insist that anyone can benefit from a new haircut, a good shave at the hands of your barber, and whatever your gender, never be afraid to seek out a certified Esthetician for a facial, pedicure, or manicure.

It really is down to the little things.

Getting a manicure or pedicure is a treat, but it can also be a chore. Always book for a service when you feel well and want to be social.
Don't EVER be tempted to go to the unlicensed strip mall salons to combat time or price. The hygiene standards are generally atrocious, and training is poor and uninformed. Of course in many US States licensing is a legality, which I absolutely applaud. If it's just a polish color change that you need then a good salon should do that without all the palaver, and often without an appointment.

You may need to be willing to wait just a little while but it can make all the difference to your day, to just to be out of the house for half an hour. You will always feel so much better if you have been pampered and have paid just a little more attention to your appearance. Not to mention the immense benefit of a little social interaction.

Cooking when sick can be a huge chore. I have learned to batch cook for when I am having a relapse. Simple meals like Chili with rice, or a

Spaghetti Bolognese can be cooked, cooled, packaged, and frozen as individual meals for days when you don't feel your best. You can buy cheap throw away containers from your local grocery store. The bonus here is that these meals are cooked from scratch, so they contain no preservatives or unpronounceable additives, to further hinder your health.

*I have put together three simple recipes which you can find at the back of this book

Housework. Yes, that!. Here is what I would suggest; Declutter.

If you have less dust collectors, then less dust will collect.
Get rid of the nik naks, put things away in cupboards, and toss the junk. There's a quick buck to be made on EBay with anything that is in good condition. It is true; One person's junk really is another person's treasure.

Invest in decent cleaning products and tools.
Swiffer do have an excellent range of products and
the results last far longer than the old spray and
cloth methods.

Keep a vacuum cleaner on each level of your home.
Lugging a cumbersome gadget up and down the
stairs really is no joke, and that alone on a day when
you feel less than your best will discourage any type
of vacuuming action.
I have a central vacuum, a Dyson AND a Roomba.
The Roomba really is priceless. Worth every cent.

Wipe the bathtub and shower down daily as you use
it. The same goes for toilets. There....Bathroom
cleaned. Keep the kitchen wiped daily and that will
alleviate the need for any big cleaning sessions.

DO the dishes EVERY day. Empty the dishwasher
EVERY day.
Piled up dishes are an awful source of frustration
and the bigger the pile becomes, the less you will be
encouraged to tackle it.

Maybe once a month you can afford to have a few
rooms cleaned professionally. If that is the case
then I absolutely recommend it. If you have
teenagers, put them to work.

As a human being you may or may not have the need for sex as part of a relationship. Every being is very different, however having a chronic illness can quickly disrupt any sex life. Whether medication is the disruptor, mobility is an issue, pain makes sex uncomfortable, or there is just a plain old loss of libido; adapting and changing your sex life can be disruptive, upsetting and frustrating...for all involved parties.

Frank discussion with your partner, your Dr. or a Councillor, perhaps all three, but whichever is best for you, will help to guide you through. Be prepared to adapt and live with drastic changes to your sex life.

They may not be changes that you want, but they may be necessary, and in some cases they may save your relationship or even a life.

Remember this; compromise and change are always better than loneliness, heartbreak or death.

Take AT LEAST one half hour daily to take a soak in the bath, have quiet time with a book, or even just to lay on the bed and relax. Switch everything off, including yourself.

If you need to let someone know that you are taking time for yourself, do so.

Then you can leave your phone in another room with the volume switched off. No TV, no radio, no kids, no spouse. Just you and total relaxation. It is possible that you could teach yourself to meditate.

I have been unsuccessful in my attempts at meditation. But I rest daily regardless.

No interruptions. No excuses.

Finally; You always need to weigh up what needs to be done, with what you would prefer to do, or what you can manage to do that day. If the TV really needs dusting, but it's a gloriously sunny day and you want to go for a walk, ALWAYS choose the walk.

The TV will still need dusting tomorrow. It really is that simple.

Education; The Most Essential Part of Living With a Chronic Illness

As a long time sufferer of chronic illness and the things that it brings to your table, you are likely to now understand what is going on with your mind, body and spirit, far better than anyone else; Including your medical team. Understanding all of what living with a chronic illness means is often a little more complex, however.

If you are recently diagnosed and have started to advocate for yourself very early in your illness, then I applaud you. You have achieved what very few of us ever manage.

Advocation at any time is a great accomplishment, especially on your own.

There may be people along your journey who will argue that they know what is best for you. Many of them will be wrong. Follow your instincts and you won't go far wrong.

Of course in this, the is the age of the internet, you have at your fingertips a wealth of knowledge and information (some good information, some less than great).

You will likely join various online support groups. Hell, you maybe even go so far as to offer advice to fellow sufferers of your disease.

Before you progress, now is a time to stop and think.

How often do you hear people who are chronically ill say "I'm single," or "I'm divorced because my partner didn't understand what I was going through." Maybe you know the person who said "I just can't cope and my friends don't call me anymore," and "I don't have anyone I can turn to." Are you one of these people?
Far too often you hear "My partner just doesn't get it'" or "My parents and kids just don't believe me."

WHY is this? The answer is so very easy.

It is one word; **EDUCATION.**

Think about it. You have been sick for many very long years. You have read this article and researched that one. You have regularly visited the GP or PCP, you have sought help from a Naturopath, Acupuncturist and Chiropractor, and you have another appointment with a new Specialist next week.

How much of this have you shared with those close to you?
Little to none, is probably the answer.
You likely live in a world that is consumed by your illness.

Your life is adjusted to work in partnership with how you feel and what you can tolerate at any given time.

Yet as you have made these adjustments, along the way you may have just forgotten to include those closest to you.

How many times has your partner sat with you at the computer with you while you Google "hives and low temperature," or "weight gain with exercise"? The answer is likely never, because they are probably at work or asleep in bed, while you type frantically at your computer, as your insomnia gives you another good ass whooping.

How many times has your partner attended a Dr. appointment with you?... Um never, right?

If you consider a five year chronic illness, which is what I have now lived through, that is as close as it gets to the number of years you need to be studying for and gaining a degree in medicine.

Consider next if you will how often you have spent time on the computer doing research, or time in the Drs office discussing symptoms and action plans, during that period.

How many lists and folders of symptoms, reports and clinical studies have you amassed?

Okay, so this paints a clear picture of how a chronic illness affects your life, but what about those around you?

We all know that you feel frustration, but it is also felt by those around you. Just like you they will likely feel sadness, pain, hurt, anger and perhaps even loss.
Yes, living close to someone with a chronic disease can be compared to a bereavement. The loss of the person they once knew. The death of the vibrant, outgoing and fun side of the partner that they chose to spend their life with. This does not mean that this is your fault, nor should you be blamed in any way, but you can help them to understand by involving them in learning about your illness.

You must consider though, is this what they signed up for? You sure as hell didn't.
What if the tables were turned.... Could you live with someone who was chronically sick, like you are?

At this point the picture should be much clearer! Just this short explanation really puts a new perspective on things, doesn't it?

Those around you cannot possibly understand how you feel. That is a crazy notion.
Yet you continually ask yourself this; "Why don't they understand? Why don't they believe me?"

First; they don't live it. They live near it. They
cannot possibly understand.
Second; they are not well educated in the matters of
chronic illness...if at all.
You must help them to become educated.

We all know of an illness called Cancer. We all know
that it makes you very sick, and it can be terminal.
Of course we are aware of these facts, because we
hear about them all the time. We are all somewhat
educated about what causes it and how to try to
prevent it, but whoever heard of Hashimoto's
Thyroiditis, Lyme Disease or Cushing's Disease?
Right?
All of these and many more, can also cause varying
levels of illness, and sometimes they can cause
death.
But who knew?

Unfortunately, many chronic diseases are
considered invisible. There is no physical
abnormality and therefore others assume that

because you look "fine" that there is nothing wrong with you.

In trying to explain this to someone who is finding it hard to understand, perhaps you could compare what you feel to a headache, muscle spasms or a toothache. Many of us have experienced this at some point in time and none of these are visible, but we all believe it when someone says they are having such an experience.

As the owner of a chronic illness, it can be very difficult to communicate how and what you are feeling.

So often Drs. will tell you that you are "just" depressed, or that you have Fibromyalgia,* the most recent diagnosis for a chronic illness that your Dr. cannot figure out, or is too incompetent or lazy to investigate. You believe this, because it's what your Dr. tells you, he is after all; the expert.
Your Dr. may then push some pain and anti-depression pills, and write you off. I know this happens because a Dr. I was attending told me as much, just before he tried to accuse me of shopping for pain medication.

On this occasion I was quick to point out to the Dr. that I was happy to live without pain medication, if he could just give me an explanation or a diagnosis for my symptoms and illness. I still only take pain medications perhaps twice weekly, and I never accepted a later offer from the very same Dr. for opioids, which he wanted to prescribe so that I would be able to "exercise pain free"...

Eventually some of you win through. Through discussion with others like yourself, through research, through sheer bloody mindedness and a strong will to not only survive, but you will thrive, you will come to a place where you are in control. A place where you have such a good understanding of the situation you are in, that you are able to communicate with confidence to your medical team. You learn to question decisions by your Dr. and you even offer up suggestions of your own on how your treatment should progress.

Along the way, would it not make sense to share this knowledge and understanding with those close to you? Family and friends...perhaps even colleagues, if you are still lucky enough to be able to work.

It is not however, a good idea to constantly tell your family what hurts, how bad the pain in your head is, or how many times you threw up today. Especially if these folk are involved in your care and somewhat already understand the situation. If you have a need to constantly reinforce the fact that you feel unwell, this is likely borne of a need for attention, and probably needs to be addressed by your medical team. You really can and should learn to deal with your illness in a much more positive manner.

If your family isn't involved in your care, then by all means explain to them how you feel on a day to day basis. Tell them that changes and even remission can happen. Explain your worst day and your best. Provide them with a few good honest pieces of literature. I'm writing this book just for that very reason.

Establish some guidelines. Rules if you will, for the wellbeing of everyone involved.

In choosing to educate those around you, a primary discussion is critical. A meeting of minds.

A real conversation about how everyone concerned feels. You must find out where everyone stands as early as possible after diagnosis or onset of symptoms. If there is no understanding and no communication, there becomes an instability, things can quickly become unbalanced, and it's a given that nine out of ten times a listing ship will sink.

Express to your partner or your parents, to your children, and your close friends, that you want to have a more productive and active life, but if that is to happen then "this is what we need to do to make it work."
If your partner is invested in your relationship at all, they will inevitably open up and offer some insight into how they feel too. This will probably be a very emotional time, but you will go on to feel so much relief.

If your partner keeps a closed shop then you will need to be proactive, ask them what their frustrations are, ask what they need to know about your illness. Share the relevant information that you have gathered. Draw pictures or make an easy to understand graphic, if that's what it takes. Use trusted self help websites, or social media forums. Pose questions to chat room allies to gain insight and further educate yourself.

When sharing knowledge you can make up a simple list. Bullet point your symptoms on a list, and if you know why those symptoms are occurring you can write a short explanation next to it. Go through this with your partner and family and allow them to ask questions.

Imagine a scenario that has likely been happening for a long time;

Your partner comes home from work after a long, hectic and frustrating day and asks "Hi honey, how are you?" Do you focus on the positive and say; "I read two chapters from that book by Erica Worth today, they provided me with some useful information"?

It's very likely you didn't say that, but that will always sound better than "I felt like shit all day, so I went back to bed." Which is what you actually told them!

If you start to focus on the positive, it will quickly lessen any tension, and it will help your well being too. Focus on the negative for any amount of time and it is guaranteed to make you and those around feel worse, and it WILL be destructive in the long run.

It's okay to have an off day and to feel sorry for yourself from time to time. Everyone does it. Just don't dwell on it permanently, because it will quickly drag you all down.

It certainly is bad enough that you have to deal with the enormity of what is chronic illness.

Give those around you the tools to understand and support you in your journey, and you will not believe the changes.

Learn to work around your illness and with your family. This isn't just their education, it's also yours. If you need to nap in the afternoon but the family wants to go to the mall for the day, compromise. Nap a few hours earlier than usual and head to the mall a little later. It's likely that the mall is open until 9pm.

If there is a show you want to see, make sure the family knows you need to rest the day before, and take it easy on the day of the show. That annoying pile of laundry can wait two days.

If your partner wants to go for a walk and you tire easily, suggest an evening outing when it's cooler, and after you have rested.

Stand in the backyard and watch the Aurora Borealis at 1am. You are awake anyway and it really is spectacular!

Make exclusive time for your partner, even if it's just a few hours weeding the yard as the sun comes up.

If you feel good, be spontaneous. You may be tired the next day, but you will learn to adjust accordingly.

Give your partner space. Just because someone is not at work, it doesn't mean they have to spend all their free time with you. If you give a partner the space they need to breathe and think, it's likely to bring them closer to you.

Learn that nothing is as important as your happiness and the happiness of those around you, but to get to that place everyone must be educated, and learning is a constant process, so you must all be a work in progress.

Life is one long learning experience and education is key.

*Fibromyalgia is a relatively new and often controversial illness, only recently recognized as a stand alone illness in the US. There are no blood tests or scans that can be considered when giving a diagnosis, merely tender points on the body, and

Drs. will readily tell you that they don't really understand what it is.

Many Drs. still do not believe that it exists as a stand alone illness. Yet many people are diagnosed and it is often a misdiagnosis. I personally know people who have been misdiagnosed with fibromyalgia, only to later be told that they have thyroid illness, adrenal disruption, arthritis, PCOS, and even MS. These are people who are well educated and have been mislead and mistreated.

I am one of those people, and I can assure you that when my medication is optimal the "fibromyalgia" vanishes into thin air.

I could write an entire chapter on fibromyalgia the monster, myth and legend, but for now I will leave you with this. Fibromyalgia is a diagnosis that is easy for your Dr. and will save him an awful lot of time and effort. It is often comes with a vague generalization, and for the most is left uninvestigated and untreated.

I will at this time leave it to your better judgement to best understand and further research what fibromyalgia is.

Meanwhile, you should investigate further any other symptoms that you may experience.

Visiting the Dr.

Plan A; Be prepared.
Plan B; Have a plan C, D, E and F

Many of you will immediately understand the sarcasm above. I wanted to try to be light hearted with this chapter, because I well know that Dr. visits can be one of the most frustrating and upsetting parts of being chronically ill.

If you already have a good family Physician or Primary Care Provider (PCP) who understands your illness, how to best treat that illness, and they are working in partnership with you to get you the best in medication and other help, then you are fortunate. Keep doing what you are doing and thank your lucky stars...and your Dr.
Additionally you may learn a tip or two here as well, so please feel free to read on.

Your medical care providers should always make to feel that you can always book a visit with them to discuss your symptoms as they change in any way. You should always get involved during these meetings.

This involvement can be anything from merely explaining your symptoms, to suggesting that you undergo any testing and monitoring you feel would be beneficial to your particular situation..

There should never be a limit to your involvement. This is your health....and your life.

Feel free to mention to your Dr. any literature that you may have read, and also any input from friends, family, or others you know with the same illness, if you feel that it will be beneficial input regarding your treatment. At this time it is always helpful for you to know of any family history of chronic illness, so that you can present it to your Dr. during your discussion. Your Dr. should chronicle this information electronically in your presence.

Again, if your Drs. are helpful and continue to be so, that is great.

If not, now may be a good time to move on...

In trying to find a new Dr. you should call around to all the local Drs. offices to find out whether practitioners that are accepting new clients. Book appointments with any available Drs. that you feel would be able to help you. If there is more than one

Dr. that looks like a good fit, go ahead and schedule appointments with them all. Book these appointments for a few days after you intend to see your current family practitioner.

That way if your regular Dr. is working with you, the appointments elsewhere can be cancelled.

Always be sure and be courteous when you cancel with any prospects, because you may need to revisit this option down the road, and you don't need to burn any bridges.

If however, after a visit with your current Dr. you are less than satisfied with his ability to include you in your own care, or even in his ability to actively investigate your symptoms further, and it is looking like a change of care provider may be the way to go, here is a good course of action;

Attend ALL of the pre arranged appointments and before making a final choice of Dr. Research local Practitioners online, ask friends or family for referrals, and always try to choose the Dr. who you know will treat, or who specializes in your particular illness...presuming of course that you already know what that illness is. It is advisable to ask the receptionist at the time of booking whether there is a Dr. in that office who is knowledgeable in your particular ailment.

If you are unsure of what your illness is, then it would be advisable to choose a Dr. on personal recommendations and merit.

I would always suggest that you meet with more than one prospective Dr. and make a choice after seeing them all.

When you attend the initial meeting, you should be interviewing them. Ask them questions, take time to try to figure them out, bring an advocate or ally with you to these appointments. I know this is all very time consuming and it may tire you at the time, but the final result will reap the benefits for your health because of this extra effort.

In preparation (plan A) you will need the following

A list of current medications
The date (or an approximate time of when you began to feel unwell)
A list of symptoms and possible triggers
A list of questions
A list of suggestions

You should make a request for any copies of any recent blood testing, urinalysis results, and imaging, at each appointment. Don't take no for an answer with these requests.

You are legally entitled to any and all test results pertaining to your health, and a decent practitioner will happily oblige.

Remember this is YOUR health. You are more than entitled to copies of any notes and records, and you are equally as entitled to make suggestions regarding treatments. You can ask any questions you feel relevant regarding medications and referrals.

Do at least a little research on your symptoms and or illness and arm yourself with some basic knowledge before each visit. Challenge your Dr. a little, this is a good way to find out if he really knows what he is talking about.

Try to dress smartly for your appointments. I know that sounds a little odd, but some Drs. can be a little snobby and judgemental. If you dress smartly, you are less likely to be considered a flake...Yes, really.

I have tested this theory and it is absolutely correct, but I also discovered that you risk looking "well" if you look "nice." I have had to point out to my Dr. that just because I look nice, it doesn't stop the pain I am experiencing, and looking nice is a huge boost to my confidence, when dealing with the agony and disruption that my illness brings.

Take an advocate with you to medical appointments whenever possible.
Preferable is a family member or a close friend who is aware of the fine details of your illness. With extra ears and eyes in the office, a Dr. is likely to treat you more respectfully, and explain things in more detail.

Take written notes, or record your meetings on your smartphone.

If the Dr. is reluctant to allow recording or to give you copies of your records, respectfully remind him that you are legally entitled to the information, as it is about you.
If reluctance shines through, perhaps mention that your legal representative advised you that it is well

within your rights to gather this information for your personal records.

Perhaps ask the Dr. what he would do in your situation. How would they expect to be treated, or how they would like their spouse to be treated if they were very ill? No need for rudeness, but you can be a little challenging.

Plans B and C may become necessary at this time....

If your Dr. is steadfast and unwilling to involve you in your treatment plan, or even to give you access to your own records, it may be time to move on.

I speak from experience when I say this can be extremely draining, very upsetting, and incredibly time consuming.

It may take years to make the positive changes that you need. You may be discouraged and upset, and that is natural and understandable, but please persevere on your path.
It is so worth that time and effort.

I now have a team of Drs. who are all willing to discuss and disclose. They know that I am my own advocate because I have told them so. They have all thanked me for being proactive, informed, and challenging.
This is the result I persevered for and that I absolutely deserved. You deserve no less.
Two of these Drs are even happy to learn from me. A great result all around.

Keep in mind, in any new relationship you should start as you mean to go on. Be assertive and confident, but not abrasive or confrontational. Collect notes right from the first meeting and continue to share your ideas and make suggestions. You will feel a difference just by having a team you can count on and work with.

Specialists and Consultants

During the progression of your care, there may be
need for a referral to a Specialist or Consultant.
Your Primary Care Practitioner or Dr. will perhaps
suggest this, alternately you may specifically
request this service, especially if you have been
given the name of a reputable Consultant.
Either way, you will need to be prepared.

Between the time that you visit your Dr. to request a
referral and the initial visit to the Specialist, there
are a few things that you should do, that will greatly
increase your chances of success in formulating a
care plan at the Consultant's office.

Keep a journal; make notes as frequently as you can,
or you feel the need to. Document all changes to
your health and any factors that surround you;
changing weather, pain levels, medications, diet,
exercise and any stressors. Make a comprehensive

list of your current medications and active symptoms.

You will likely have this information filed from your first visit with your PCP, and you should utilize this information as often as you need to. Make any adjustments as necessary, and reuse this document, it can save you so much time and effort.
Be very aware of what your Primary Care Provider writes in his letter to the Consultant.
If you are unaware of the content contained in the referral, it can really have an impact on how the Consultant treats you and your illness.
Forewarned really is forearmed.
You NEED that referral information so that you can educate yourself on how your illness can progress, how it is treated, periods of remission, and how to best discuss the care plan and medications you may need.
Have a frank discussion with the Specialist and don't allow him to fob you off or treat you like you are under educated.

Yes, Consultants are specially trained, but they do not live with these afflictions and illnesses, so their insight however well meaning and tailored, is usually gained from textbooks and ten minute bedside visits with patients who they maybe see once or twice.

The Consultant is not living with the illness and you most certainly are.
Share your experiences with them, in the hope to gain insight into your condition and perhaps further add to their education.
Don't be afraid to insist on further investigation, testing and medication, if you feel it is required to aid your situation.

If you have a bad experience with a Consultant, revisit your PCP promptly and tell him about that experience. Request a second opinion with another Specialist. It is your legal right, and if your PCP is fighting your corner he will agree right away.
You may also lodge a formal complaint about a PCP, nurse or any other practitioner if their behaviour warrants doing so. Put in writing a complaint to

your local Physicians (or respective) governing body.

You may not get the answers you require, but they must keep a record of any complaints about members, and if more people take that initiative eventually your voice will be heard.

I have had to request second opinions with new Consultants twice. I have made three formal complaints about Drs. and I changed my PCP in 2012 after he laughed at me when I requested thyroid testing, right before insisting I was just depressed and obese.
It's not easy thing to have to do, it can leave you feeling deflated and stupid. It can also strip you of any confidence you had. You can be made to feel troublesome and as though you are wasting time and resources. I can assure you that is not the case, and I would urge you to continue to insist upon the care that you absolutely deserve.

Remind yourself that this is exactly the course of action that the Dr. you are visiting would take were he in your position, and you deserve no less than the best that your care team can offer.

You will rue the day if you settle for less than the best, yet you will rejoice in the results if you continue to fight, to advocate for your your health...your life.

Remission and Relapse

Sometimes, during a chronic illness, you will find yourself feeling quite well; "Tip Top.' or "On Form," if you will.
It's possible you will regain physical strength. You may be vibrant, clear thinking and task oriented. You may resume physical activities, social engagements and hobbies.

This really is not a bad thing. This is great, but I'd like to advise caution before attempting anything with any vigor and here's why;

When I started working out in the latter months of 2015, after many years of not having the energy or even the inclination to climb two flights of stairs on most days, I rejoined the local network of gyms. With my husband by my side, I embarked upon a one hour workout, fifteen minute stretch or yoga session, and fifteen minutes of gentle aquacise; three times a week.

My workouts alternated between seated elliptical or static bike and a gentle weight routine.

NOTE that in my teens I took three; two hour karate classes each week. One; two hour ballroom dancing class, and I rode my horse at least four times a week, for two or more hours. I kept a field and stable clean, and I rode my bicycle twenty miles on a Saturday.

It's not like I came from a sedentary background, yet getting back into the gym was a huge accomplishment, especially considering my health of late.

So I made my return and I was going great guns. I even ventured into the gym on a third and fourth day some weeks. I managed to be in regular attendance for three months, missing only two sessions.

I'm not going to lie. I often felt like I had been beaten the next day, but I figured that it was improving my strength and fitness, so I persevered. I felt extremely proud of myself, hell, I even treated myself to a gym specific cell phone case and new workout clothes.

Then I got an infection. ANOTHER bloody infection. I had swollen glands all over the back of my head and neck, for which I have still no diagnosis. This infection came with fever, body and facial swelling, pain and malaise. In fact it caused an episode of TOTAL exhaustion.
This is very common with a Lupus diagnosis, but it drives me to total distraction.

This latest "flare" put me out of action completely for three weeks, right down to not being able to complete any cooking and cleaning. The first week of those three, I spent a fun filled time in the bathroom after taking just three pills, from a ten day course of antibiotics.
I took no more antibiotic pills after that third one.

My Dr. ran my C Reactive Protein (inflammatory marker) and it was up to twenty. This is much higher than it should be as "normal" is considered to be under ten, but this was not a surprise to me. I could feel it. I could see it.

My T3 and T4 (Thyroid) were both registering on the low side, even when I was taking 210 mg Natural Desiccated Thyroid daily. They are still registering as low.
I was adding Vitamin D3 at 10,000 units daily and additional Ferritin (Iron).
I was adding Cinnamon to help level my blood sugar and Theracurmin for inflammation. Yet still everything was unbalanced.
Of course I had researched the pros and cons of any supplements before adding them to my regimen.

It turned out that my thyroid levels were not the only unstable hormones I had either. My Estrogen was high and Progesterone and Testosterone were registering low.
My Thyroid antibodies were high and my A1C was on the rise, suggesting that my insulin resistance was increasing. I had markers for a Streptococcus infection, but the origin was unknown.

For three months after this recent relapse, I was still struggled with my spelling and speech. I was jumbled and confused, I couldn't think of the words to describe things.
My memory had taken a small beating.

Okay, so you've read all of this, you are probably thinking "So what, you got an infection, what is the relevance of all this?"

The relevance is this; This was a huge warning to me, to minimise my physical activities and watch closely for physical and mental signs that say just that. Some may be minute signs, but they will be there.

If any part of your body is feeling like it's been beaten, you should listen to it. I didn't listen, but I should have. My body was absolutely saying "don't push yourself too hard and stop trying to impress yourself or anyone else."
I hadn't tried to impress anyone else in at least three years before this. I had already worked out that my well being was much more important than an entire world full of other people. Perhaps I let myself forget that by pushing so hard at the gym.

Don't get me wrong I was enjoying really my
workouts and I attend the gym once again now that
I feel much recovered, but now I am so very very
aware of overworking and burning out.

As quickly as you can regain pseudo composure and
normality, my experience is a sign that you can be
back in the doldrums twice as quick.
After all, when was the last time any of us with a
chronic illness actually felt 100% normal, Okay or
well ? Our highs are considerably less great than
someone who is not, or never has been ill.
I was starting to feel very low during my latest
crash. I mean sad, unhappy, depressed almost,
feeling which I had not experienced since I had
commenced my Natural Desiccated Thyroid, and Bio
Identical Hormone medication in March 2013.

I know now that by overworking myself I had
unstabilized my medication, which threw my
immune system out of whack, at which point my
endocrine levels were unbalanced, my thyroid
antibodies levels were elevated, and I had
increasingly high levels of inflammation.

As I wrote that I visualized a big line of dominoes,
just falling, one after the other, after the other.
Keep that imagine in mind for if you ever over exert.

To help me with my recovery, the medicine I was taking as a sedentary person, has now had a total re-evaluation. I quickly completed the bloodwork to re-evaluate my levels, and I attended an appointment with my Bio Identical Hormone team in late March 2016. It took over a month for some of the blood panels to be returned, so there was some waiting in limbo, and of course then came the $350 fee!

I know I'm not invincible, but I was feeling hopeful that I may be on the right track, that the exercise was increasing my endorphins, metabolic rate and natural hormone output, therefore aiding my recovery.

What I learned was that I need to track and adjust my panels very carefully when adding or decreasing activity, and I'd advise anyone in a similar situation to do the same.

I also realized, perhaps for the first time, that my endocrine system is broken, and will likely never recover fully, hence the need for medications to begin with. It seems that I had been in denial for sometime.

I quickly found out was that I was pushing too hard on the leg raises and I had probably taken one too many visits to the Steam Room; which incidentally can be a playground for virus and bacteria of all descriptions. Give the germs a compromised immune system and they will be all over it.
This was a huge personal learning curve.
Fortunately this time it was just that and not something more serious.
Let's call it an educational experience, something to be noted and learned from. A minor bump in the road. During those 3 weeks of total inability, with feelings of weakness and failure, I felt like the road roller trying so very hard to resurface that very road, was actually a jack hammer breaking me apart.

I'm back in the gym now. Okay, I'm on a decreased work out plan, but I'm feeling much improved, full of positivity, and now I'm aware of the signs to slow or temporarily rest, I will be taking full advantage of knowing them.

However invincible you feel today, you should always limit your activities and engagements. Level out. Take at least a day to recover after each session of physical activity or social outing.

It's this simple; Don't try and lift 200 lbs and run a marathon, when you can't even stand up without pain first thing in the morning.

Listen to your body; go with your gut. If you are feeling off, weak, or less than able, that is your human mechanism telling you to slow it the heck down!
Do enough to stabilize and maintain, increase if you feel able. If you feel less than able then you should take a break, regain your composure, reevaluate and restructure.

It's all about give and take; being able when you can, and not about forcing yourself both physically and mentally, when you clearly cannot.

Discuss with the qualified staff at your gym and your healthcare team before undertaking any kind of exercise, as it can be very dangerous to exert yourself when living with certain diseases. If you are given the all clear to work out put a plan into place. Revisit your goals regularly.
Remember, even a simple walk around the block will be beneficial to some of us.

Your current self feeling ok, is always better than your future self feeling beaten and broken.

Learning to Live with a Change of Self Image

I was very slim until the age of seventeen, fluctuating between 112lb. and 120lb. at at a height of five feet six inches. I guess I physically presented as what western society would consider attractive. At around the age of nineteen I gained weight. It wasn't a huge amount of weight, but enough that I could tell the difference, as could those around me. In less than a year I then lost that weight and in the twenty-five years since I turned twenty years old, I have gained and lost...Gained and lost....GAINED and gained. Then with a recent adjustment in my medication, I lost again.

My most recent loss was small, but we should also count the one half inch off my height.

At times over the years, I felt that I needed to join dieting groups to control my unexplainable gains. I rarely lost more than 10 lb this way even through months of dieting.
At other times the weight would simply evaporate and I would become almost gaunt.

Here is where I have to point out that never once did I change my eating habits or my lifestyle during these losses and gains.

Of course, I am well aware now at the age of forty-five that this has all been the fault of my broken, unstable and ill balanced endocrine system, topped off with a side of autoimmune disease. The thought never goes away that had I been tested regularly, completely, or for different illnesses, by my family Dr. when I was younger, I would have perhaps been able to control better, that which has caused me to be at a weight of 235lb. now.
This is not my heaviest. At one point I weighed in at 260lb.

During the time since diagnosis (and before that with many symptoms) I have had to deal with mild to severe attacks of acne, hair loss, hirsutism (dark, thick facial or body hair) and edema (swelling).

These are just a few of the physical issues and challenges that I have faced.

All of these physical changes make a person look very different and;

When people look different, others can be very judgmental.

When others judge you, it can be crippling to your confidence.

When your confidence is low it can drastically change the way you live and behave.

Do you see what just occurred there?
In just three short steps life can become unbearable.

You become lost, hopeless, depressed and demoralized.

It takes no time at all to quickly become a vicious cycle.

The weight issue especially has had many differing effects on my self confidence, and there have been times when I have been miserable, sad, and even clinically depressed about my changed appearance.

Not so now though.

I have, on the journey through learning about my conditions, and through being judged unfairly and unnecessarily by those who have no business in my business, learned to embrace myself once again.

I have learned that there are many others out there just like me. Some have not yet been as lucky, they cannot come to terms with who they are now that illness has become the major part of their life. I hope this book will help those of you that feel this way.

Many of you already have taken control of the way you portray and believe in yourselves, and those are often the first steps in feeling well or at least improved.

These will be the first steps in regaining you. Maybe not the you of previous times, but the newly educated, tolerant, beautiful, vibrant, patient, understanding and sharing; you.

We all must learn that we are not here to please others. Even those of us who are not unwell sometimes need to learn this.

We must each learn to please ourselves before we devote our time and energy to others.

Selfishness is a huge part of feeling well and becoming confident. It can take a while, and progression can be slow, but if you can grasp the idea that being selfish is not at all selfish, the rest is fairly plain sailing.

Learn to say no to others. Go for a nap if you need to. Heck, go for a nap if you want to. Eat a bar of chocolate. Watch cartoons in bed until noon. Wear whatever you want. Color your hair blue, or pink, or green. Lay in bed for two hours after the alarm goes off. Go to Mexico or Las Vegas for a week on your own...I did. Stay in your pajamas all weekend. Travel. Get a tattoo... I know a few superb tattooists who would be honored to ink you up.
All of these things are so simple; but you need them. You need to do them, and other things like them. They will help you discover, or rediscover, who you are, and what is your (new) purpose.
If you go out and you hear another person discussing your appearance, feel free to let them know that how you present yourself is absolutely not their business. Ask them why it is any of their business? Question their right to judge. It is so very liberating and empowering to not have to conform to any other person's ideals and standards. NEVER should you feel the need to justify your appearance

or (law abiding and decent) behavior to others. Nor should you tolerate any manner of abuse from others.

 Once you have come to the understanding that you are you and no-one can take that away from you, whether you have gained weight, need help with mobility, if you have memory lapses, or you cannot be as social as you once were.....

Once you find peace with who you are at this moment, you will find it so much easier to find who you want to be in the very near future.
If that means not looking in the mirror, or sitting in front of it for an hour at a time, so be it. Do whatever makes you feel confident and in control.

Just be you. It's that easy.

Managing Pain

Pills and Alternatives

I'm not aware of any chronic illness that does not come without pain on some level, but I know this for certain; pain on any level can be debilitating, demoralizing and life changing.

I am one of the unfortunate ones. I live with at least some form of mild pain every day of my life.

It is never in a specific place and it can be burning, achy, throbbing, stabbing and shooting; all at the same time, individually...or intermittently. It can be widespread or concentrated in just a small area. It can appear rapidly, or slowly over the course of the day.

Some days I can function exceptionally well and carry out everything I need to accomplish, or more. Other days I am almost totally immobile. Of course I prefer the former.

Pain is all encompassing and can include, but is not confined to; headaches, muscle pain, bone stiffness and tenderness, cramping, stomach disturbances, infections, hematoma, skin irritations and skin lesions.

If left unmanaged pain can quickly lead to depression, fatigue, and immobility, which will only serve to complicate your illness further.

Depression is in itself a separate and very serious issue, and while I have lived with several episodes of depression, it really is something I won't discuss at this time, as I feel it needs to be addressed professionally, and it absolutely needs to be dealt with promptly in each and every case.

My depression paled into the distance almost as soon as my hormone issues started being addressed correctly. Almost thirty years of living with anxiety and depression in some form...miraculously gone.

I cannot speak to each of your cases as far as depression, but I can absolutely say that it is very rare that an episode of depression just disappears, and I would strongly advise that you seek professional help for anything that you feel is more than unhappiness or general sadness.

In dealing, coping, and living with pain, we must consider many things.
First and most important is our own self worth, our well being.

Consider always when dealing with differing levels of pain; any adjustment in your daily schedule, circumstances, habitat, weather, diet, stressors, medications, and exercise.

After I considered these things and tailored my life to allow me to live in the best way I could with my illness, it enabled me to work around, and with my pain. It is not always a pleasant experience, but I feel it is certainly the most beneficial one.

Try compromises and readjustments..as many readjustments as are necessary, to get to the place you need to be at.

Discuss with your medical team right away if you are not able to manage any reasonable routine without pain being a major factor.
Take a little time each day to relax and reevaluate. Be aware always. Use your journalling to make connections and realizations for why any pain may increase or subside.

I rarely take pain medication during the day and I might take it twice a week at night if I really cannot relax. The reason for this is that I would rather feel something, than be unaware and unable to function on some level, any level.

Pain medications can quickly become a necessary evil if you are not aware of how best to take them.

Be very aware of how easy it can be to become reliant on medications, while making absolutely no improvements in your living standards or the management of any pain you experience, yet falling quickly into addiction.

I have a teenager in the home who already has to deal with me being unable to do certain things at times. I'm certainly not going to then expose her to an addicted and absent parent, just because I am too ignorant, uneducated, or too lazy to monitor and manage my pain.

I'm absolutely not saying that you shouldn't take the medication the Dr. prescribes you. I would advise however that you consider very carefully what is a good practice, and what isn't. Agree to a pain management plan with your medical team. Follow the rules, and immediately report changes in pain levels, resistance to medications, and the ability to function well. Don't wait until you are past the point of no return.

That is just adding yet another level of illness to something you are already struggling with.

We all know that is it just easier to medicate than to work towards improvement, or maintaining a better lifestyle? Are you taking the easy way out, or are you worth more than that? Are willing to work towards taking the high road? I think you are so worth that effort.

My pain is all over the place, so even when I am unmedicated, I can go from a very high level of pain, to virtually none several times over the course of a day. Often the pain recurs in a different place than it was, earlier that day...
I'll take that pain every time, over a day of total unawareness and an inability to perform on any level.

I do feel that heat helps to relieve my pain immensely, and I often visit the local gym to use the steam room, sauna and hot tub if my pain levels are high.

This is great for a little light socializing too. Add a little light stretching in the hot tub and you'll notice a difference right away.

A tissue or two dipped in paraffin wax and placed on localized areas is always beneficial. Hospitals would use this method in the 80's and 90's, and you can now buy a small paraffin wax heater from any drugstore for around $100.

In utilizing this method you must always be wary of burning.

Aromatherapy administered correctly can also be immensely helpful. Essential Oils must be used according to the labels and you must always check for allergies and contraindications before starting a regimen. A visit to a certified Aromatherapist is advised.

Diffusers and candles are a less expensive alternative to oils and are readily available and easy to use, so that you are able to treat yourself to an hour "me time" at least once a week. Light the candle, close the curtains, switch off any electronics, lay on the bed and concentrate on you and only you. Just the fact that any stressors are away and forgotten for an hour can help to ease any pain and tension.

Epsom salts in a bathtub of well heated water, with a candle burning on the counter and the bathroom lights dimmed, is a rather decadent way to help ease all over body pain. It is proven to work and it is easily accessible. Salts are around $10 for a large bag in most drug stores in North America. The magnesium in the salts is known to be beneficial especially for pain from arthritis. Magnesium deficiency in North Americans can be linked to high rates of stroke, osteoporosis, arthritis, digestive disturbance and chronic fatigue among other illnesses. Of course an oral supplement can also be helpful, but is not nearly as pleasant as my scenario.

If you have mobility issues and difficulties getting in and out of the tub, arrange to have help available for when you need it, and seriously consider installing an aid, or a walk in tub. Consult with your insurer to see if you qualify for assistance when buying these things.

Always consider trying natural alternatives as apart of your pain management plan, before you resort to synthetic medications. Discuss this option with your Dr. You may be very pleasantly surprised. Research local Naturopaths and Practitioners. Ask your friends for referrals.
Most Canadian Insurance companies cover up to $500 in a twelve month period for each of the following and at times additional practitioners;

Massage
Acupuncture
Chiropractor

Take a little time to research when finding a practitioner. Newly trained, or less well trained people can be more of a hindrance than a help, and will quickly suck up your insurance allowance.

Living with pain and tolerating it, while being functional and alert, is often a compromise that you will have to make.

On the flip side you may have a life of nonfunctioning and addiction.

Choose carefully

Diet and Exercise

We touched briefly on exercise in the chapter on relapse, but changes in diet and the addition of a little exercise really do warrant a little more discussion, because adjusting and tailoring these things can drastically improve your situation.

Obviously some of you with illnesses such diabetes, insulin resistance, and Crohn's will absolutely know your restrictions when it comes to diet.

Those of you with physical disabilities such as MS, Parkinson's and arthritis, may not even be able to manage a short daily walk, but any small challenge can be beneficial, and if you are having a day where you feel able to add a little exercise, it is always worth at least attempting to take the challenge, so read on anyway...

As someone who needs to be wary of what I eat, and who suffers from varying levels of pain; chronic to very mild; and often in minutes, I can only tell you how I incorporate a little extra exercise into my own routine, and I can offer an insight into how it can be really easy and seem like little or no effort..on some days at least!

I try to shop for food every day or so, this helps to ensure that my food is fresh, and I don't have much waste. This method also allows me to buy fresh produce which is often reduced in price. I am able to eat a more varied and less, or non processed diet, by shopping this way.

I try very hard to avoid processed sugars.
The Bi-daily shop also means that I get a short walk every other day or so, as I cover the entire grocery store. I try to complete all the aisles, even when I know I won't need anything from them, which makes my walk last about 30-40 minutes. I try to avoid canned or packaged goods, and my trips really are just about being out and about.

In addition to my autoimmune and endocrine ailments, I suffer with infrequent and random stomach disturbances, which have been diagnosed by my Dr. as Irritable Bowel Disease, but this has never been investigated. As a result of this I often feel far safer walking in a place that I know has a washroom. Walks in the park are great, but there are times when they are a little unpredictable as far as visiting the restroom is concerned!

Only recently did it become apparent that my cortisol levels were rising as a result of over exercise and this was not aiding my weight loss, yet further impeding it. Not only was I not losing weight, but I would exercise intensely for an hour or so I would then suffer agonizing pain for the next two or three days as a result of the raised, and rapidly dropping cortisol levels.

This all became apparent after my last big flare in early 2016, after an infection, which I also mentioned in my chapter on relapse and remission.

I eventually realized I could incorporate gentle exercise into my daily routine.
I still swim at least twice a week and I use a treadmill, elliptical, and gentle weights, when I feel

the urge, but I absolutely don't bust a gut to become Mrs Universe any more

SO; you already know about my supermarket walks...

On days when I feel I can, here's what I do, and you probably can too;

Instead of one trip into the basement to take laundry I do three trips. Another three trips when I go to put the clothes away.

I will walk around the house twice if I need to go to a certain room. Fortunately the design of my house makes that possible. The fact that I forget many times why I'm going into a room, often gives me an added lap!

If I'm cooking and I require three pans from a drawer, I make three separate trips to the drawer.

If there is a bag of garbage and a bag of vegetable waste to take outside, I take them separately. It's all about expending just a little a little more energy.

It's just small stuff, but it all helps.

I wear a Samsung Gear watch to track my steps and adding the extra effort adds on third more steps in my daily routine.

Some days doing these simple tasks increases my fatigue and pain and so I rest. Some days simple tasks don't hurt and I do my extra steps. I know my limits and I work within them, if I ever need to stop and rest I do.

You will soon learn what your limits are.

If you are able, willing and have the time available; At a cost of around one dollar a day you can have at your disposal an entire network of gyms. My local County recreation membership gives me access to five different indoor facilities and two outdoor facilities.

That's three swimming pools and many wellness centres, plus several outdoor workout areas.

Whatever your illness, you must always discuss with with a Dr. and a certified personal trainer before attempting any workout regimen.
Have your Dr. write, advising your trainer of your limits and goals.

Once you have established a routine you should start slowly and work thoroughly, but remember that you don't have to attend a session if you feel unwell, tired or have other social engagements.
This is about your well being, and sometimes that means doing less.

To help balance my diet I bought a juicer, and I have been very impressed with the many combinations that I can produce. I try to stay away from fruits that are too sweet and I will only have one small glass of fruit juice daily, but just that one glass can stop any hunger pangs and can help to balance blood sugar levels if you have any type of insulin imbalance.
Of course vegetables can be used in a juicer too, but I prefer my vegetables lightly steamed or raw and crunchy!

You can find an almost infinite number of juicer recipes online.

For those of you who like the vegetable juices, you could likely drink two or three glasses a day to curb hunger and help to balance your metabolism.

If you encounter cravings allow yourself two pieces of chocolate or perhaps a cup of hot chocolate, as an alternative to an entire bar of chocolate or five cookies. Pickles and a few saltines for those that need a savory kick. Again, a glass of water can often help to fill you up before any snacking.

Going on a road trip? Try taking snacks with you on trips away from the house in a small resealable sandwich bag; baby carrots, bell pepper, melon, apples and cucumber slices can stop you from pulling in at the gas station and buying a chocolate bar, or heading for the nearest fast food outlet!

Even a simple homemade sandwich is better than a sugary donut or a granola.

Just by giving yourself an five extra minutes to prepare these foods you can make big changes.

Portion size and regular meals are definitely something to consider changing.

Add fifty percent more vegetables and reduce rice, potato or pasta servings by the same amount, and you will generally see a physical change in a matter of weeks.

Using a smaller plate is often all it takes to make the difference in reducing portion size.

Drinking a glass of water about 20 minutes before you eat a meal will help you to stay hydrated and make you feel less hungry.

Eating at four hour intervals will help to keep your insulin levels and blood sugars balanced. I have found that doing this really helps me to curb any cravings and minimizes stomach disturbances.

Again, consider making a batch of Chili, Cottage pie, or Bolognese*, to freeze in individual servings. You can always use chicken or turkey as an alternative to ground beef. This method is superb if I you are often in a hurry, or you just don't feel like cooking because of a relapse. The only work involved is to take the food from the freezer to defrost and then reheat. No messing and no mess. All the ingredients were fresh and there are no preservatives or additives. Cost effective and so much better for you than store bought, pre packaged foods.

*Recipies at the back of this book

None of this information is rocket science. It may seen like a hassle on paper, but life is much easier when you are in control and organized, and it makes so much sense when this information is all put into action. Changes always take some time to adjust to, but they really can become the norm, and you will see some very positive changes as a result of these adaptations.

Journaling and Scheduling

Journaling is ABSOLUTELY the most effective way of tracking any changes and symptoms pertaining to your illness. That does not mean you should be obsessively writing down everything you do, feel and say. You will quickly learn what needs to be noted, and what is okay to ignore.

I find the best way to journal is when something significant changes.
Most recently I have been getting up in the night to pee more than once. I recorded this as it was a significant change, and so it needed to be logged.

I noted this because it hasn't happened in a while, though it has happened for prolonged periods several times before. It seems to only happen when my cortisol levels are lower and my pain levels are generally much increased. I won't necessarily go to the Dr. right away as I know why it happens, but it is helpful to have the information on file, and then I can compare patterns or occurrences.

When I get prolonged periods of pain, or I am unable to do something one day that I could do the day before, I will always journal those things.
If I manage to go a full day without a nap, I journal it. Today is not that day!

You will learn to use whatever medium is more comfortable for recording data. A pen and paper, cellphone, notebook or laptop. It is advisable to always backup your records. You may quickly find a pattern emerging when you have a hard copy to view, and that record could be quite important as part of your recovery or treatment.

Whenever you visit the Dr. be they new to you, or in it for the long haul, make a note. Bullet point what you discussed; any new progress, steps backwards, or regimen changes. This can be very helpful as a guide, and can be great in comparing visits and the progression of any plan.

Does the weather make a difference to your state of mind, or cause physical changes?
You may never notice if you don't keep track.

How about changes to diet, levels of exercise, or medication increases and reductions? Taking medications just a few hours early or late may make a very significant difference to the way you feel, or your symptoms.

If you are regularly recording that very valuable information, you will notice very quickly if changes are happening for a specific reason.

It could really make a big difference to your treatment plan and your ability to thrive while living with your disease.

If you decide to try massage, chiropractor treatments, acupuncture or Reiki treatments along with your care regimen, or even just as a one off treatment, be sure to log any effects that this additional treatment has.

Are you more tired and forgetful at the onset of menstruation?

Does shift work cause changes that you feel could be better controlled...
How about just one extra hour of sleep in the morning?

Any and all of these changes can make a massive difference to how you live, and whether you survive or thrive.

Stress can be a major factor in differing levels of malaise, depression, fatigue and pain. Stress can chronically exacerbate any symptoms. You always need to try to control any, or all stress.

Make a re-printable chart if this helps you to track. List your symptoms and check or circle them on days when things change. Note the time of day and level of pain.

Tired/energized
Pain/pain free
Mobile/immobile
Hives/clear skin
Happy/sad
Hungry/nausea

A simple smile or a sad face can show improvements or relapses.

Make it as complex or as simple as you need. If you only need to jog your memory it can be less time consuming. If you need to have more detail a chart with keywords and a short descriptive is maybe what you will need.

If journaling is something that you are successful with, perhaps scheduling is also for you.

Many of us living with illness try to accomplish everything we need to do that week in one fell swoop. It's not advisable. It often wipes us out for three of four days afterward, and then we are good for nothing. Our week is wasted.

As with the journalling, scheduling requires that leave notes on your cell, laptop, or a simple chart on the fridge. Whatever works best for you is the route to take. Trial and error may be necessary here, but you will quickly learn what is more beneficial for your particular situation.

Whatever your schedule entails, give yourself at least an hour to rest every day. Perhaps you will need two half hour breaks? I find rest is essential for me, even if my break falls between 6pm and 7pm. I NEED that break. When I rest I go to bed. I don't take my phone, I don't allow any interruptions. NO TV, radio or computer. NO stimulation whatsoever. Chances are I will have hit my wall hours before I manage to take a rest, but sometimes the needs of family do come first, and we will at times, need to allow for that.

Learn to book appointments for your hairdresser, Dr. visit, Insurance advisor, parent teacher meetings, acupuncturist etc, when you are the most alert each day. Make your schedule about YOU. It really is that easy.
My prime times are 10am-12.30pm and 5pm-8pm.

Apart from Consultant appointments, you really only need to book for everything else a day or so ahead, that way you are not bogged down and you don't start wondering "well what if I'm too tired to make it." Allow for a few easy days before any appointments, and that way you absolutely maximize the chances of getting there.

When it comes to housework, and if you are able to clean; just one room at a time can be sufficient. Don't attempt to clean the entire house at once unless you absolutely need to, or you know you will be fine afterwards.
Do one laundry load per day, dry and fold later, or another day.
If your kids are eight or older, they should be taught how to do their own chores.
Relieve your burden on yourself and teach your children some responsibility at the same time. They will thank you for it later. You will be thankful now.

Spend one half day a month bulk cooking a few simple meals. You can easily package and freeze these. Use fresh healthful ingredients.
This method is so beneficial for when you are having a busy day, or you are not doing so well. Bolognese, Shepherd's Pie and Chili with rice are so easy to bulk prepare and freeze. BALANCE in your diet is so important, and so are fresh foods and ingredients. In addition you can pre-plan your weekly meals.
This will also save you money, as you only buy the food you need.
Shopping for FRESH food each day is even better, if it fits with your schedule and capabilities.

REMEMBER, you are not doing any of this on a whim. Plan to have a seven (Or five if you don't want to include the weekends, or days off work) day chart, each day will note a few simple, but essential tasks. Give yourself a head start and a helping hand.

Overwhelmed? Don't be. All of this takes a little practice, but it is so much better than living willy nilly or day to day; pushing hard one day and then crashing for three. That is absolutely no way to live and it can impede your ability to thrive.

Journalling and scheduling will help you balance your entire life, in turn helping to keep you mentally stimulated and alert, while giving you time to concentrate on your own well being and living as close to a normal life as is likely possible.

This really is an insight into my life....

The Internet

AKA the World Wide Web...Featuring; Facebook, Google, Tumblr, Snapchat and Twitter...

All of these have place in my journey, and some of their members became my friends early in my journey with chronic illness. I use them far less now than I did when I first became very ill.

I stopped using some altogether because I have kind of figured things out in regards to my health, but when you are unable to go out and socialize because you are dog tired and in pain, any one of these forums can be a lifesaver. These online spaces can help you learn, they give you the opportunity to make friends with those similarly afflicted, and they allow you to share information with others that are looking for help or advice. The internet can make you feel worthwhile in a life where you feel like less than nothing. If you go online, you can probably get the answers you need in seconds, as opposed to waiting for months for a Dr. to answer the same question.

I totally believe that the internet can indeed lives. But be wary. The internet can also be a dark and dismal place.

I have met some great advocates for chronic illness on the web, people that I can honestly say have helped to save my life. I've had some very low points during the past five years, and some of the people who I believed were my real life friends quickly dumped me when I couldn't go out for coffee, or hook up for a BBQ. Respectively, people I never met were willing to give their time and knowledge to help me.

In return for the generosity of my online friends, I now feel that I can share my story and be an advocate for others. That is absolutely why I'm sitting right now writing these words for you.

There are a plethora of support groups and information forums on the internet. I can only advise that you are wary when joining these groups and sharing your personal information.

Some groups will prove to be priceless to you, others are less informative and may quickly ask for money. Avoid the latter. If you have verified several forums and find all of them helpful, decide which are best tailored to your needs and perhaps only subscribe to one or two, if at all. There is so much good information out there that is free. Finding it will not take you too long at all.

Never give your personal details or address to anyone online that you do not know.

You will generally be able to find links to whatever it is you are searching for, from the genuine sites that you find are useful to your situation and specific health concern. If you have a question, there will usually be someone on those sites will have an answer for you, or they will know someone else who has that answer. Use this network, but don't abuse it.

 We have all needed help, and networking can provide you with the most useful information, but use restraint and common sense when seeking guidance. Don't become a burden. Education is how we learn and grow, so don't be afraid to ask. You will often be surprised at the answers that you are given. It only takes one great answer for you to have the "AHA" moment you may need.
But if you are constantly pestering within a group, or you are making petty arguments or comments, you will quickly fall out of favor with those freely giving their time.

Be courteous always. NEVER bully, shame or abuse. Don't ever judge others. These rules apply in real life too.
You personally don't want to receive that kind of treatment, and no one else deserves it either. If someone is giving out incorrect information, politely correct them and move on.
If someone is abusive to you, simply ignore them and report them to the forum administration and ask that a moderator deals with the situation.
Don't arrange to physically meet people who you meet online on your own. If you feel it necessary to

meet a friend from the internet, then you should follow these simple steps;

Tell others about any arranged meetings, and take a friend with you.

Meet in a very public place.

Screen shot this person's profile.

Do not get into a vehicle alone with anyone you just met.

Air on the side of caution. ALWAYS.

Don't fall into the trap of trying to be there for everyone online all the time. It's not your job to solve everyone else's issues, and it can quickly bog you down and hold you back from getting yourself well. This was something that I tried to do, but it was also something that bogged me down for a while. You cannot help everyone. If you do wish to spend some time providing answers as part of a forum and you feel that it is helpful to you, schedule specific times to do so. If you see a subject on a forum that pertains to you while you are just cruising through and you have good and reliable information to share, and you can spare a little time to answer a few questions immediately, then feel free to do so. You will likely need the same attention and help at some point.

Be mindful that your time is precious and people can, and will take advantage.

DON'T start online drama. We have all seen it and some of us are previous offenders, but don't be that person; You know the one, posting the Facebook status that gives no detail other than to cause people to give them immediate attention. "Oh my god today was the worst" or "I have never felt so sick as I do now" OKAY, those of us that live as you do know that it is awful if you have very little support or you really do need help, but if that IS the case and you feel desperate, may I suggest a visit to your ER or Dr. and soon. DON'T fall into the trap of regularly trying to attract random attention online, rather drop a discreet private message to your best friend, or a close family member.

People really do quickly tire of those who constantly cry wolf. Just remember that most of us with a chronic illness know what it is like to feel isolated and alone, but we don't spend our lives posting negative or attention seeking posts. You need to learn that if you use your social networks to share music, ideas, photographs and positive experiences, your mood can lift naturally, and there will be no need to post negative statuses.

REMEMBER; the internet is not real life.

Constantly sitting at a computer or on your cell phone, can impede and retard your ability, and your inclination, to progress through your illness and indeed your life. Like everything, use the internet in moderation and use it for education and interaction, but live your life away from the screen. It is so much better for you and your health.

Beware of Charlatans

In early 2015 I was charged 775$ for a one hour appointment with an RN (Registered Nurse) who claims on her website, to have cured Addison's disease, among other things.

Was I stupid? YOU BET.
Was I desperate? More than you'll ever know.

I made this appointment with this person after seeing a different Dr. at the clinic I had been attending for 2 years. This new Dr. had told me to wear a hat and gloves in the house to help manage my very chronic pain. She had decreased medicine that I had previously been prescribed..and was feeling much better on, and then she added new synthetic medication, something that it turned out after two weeks of trying to stick with it, had awful adverse effects.
I was absolutely terrified that everything I had strived to achieve in terms of feeling well, and regaining my confidence and a partial social presence, was going to be snatched right away from me.

The nurse in the new clinic that I visited after this rather disappointing experience did no prior blood screening. Instead she used the last tests my family Dr. had ordered which were at least 4 months old. She immediately advised me to stop my Bioidentical Hormone Replacement Therapy medication. I found this odd as she was working under the guise of a BHRT practitioner. She went on to interpret all but two of those old blood tests wrong. Then she spent a whole hour not telling me much of everything that I already know, just to finally advise me I had leaky gut. I was told to consume only a blender veggie concoction for 28 days and then start to reintroduce foods one by one. I was given a poor print out of a blended juice concoction and was sent on my merry way. At this point I gained access to the private section of the clinic website. The website that gave me no more information than I could find for free online elsewhere. Of course I only found that out when I got home. This woman was about as useful as a chocolate teapot. A big old con. She even had the nerve to tell me that she herself had spent more than $30,000 trying to get well and that was why she was now practice to help others.

This woman works under the umbrella of an OB/GYN.

Who knows if the Dr. is aware of what occurs in her name? If so she is also making money for old rope and misleading some very sick people. At the time of my visit I was too caught up in my own business to even care to make a complaint. I did email the nurse and offer her a piece of my mind right away. She agreed that I shouldn't visit her again, but offered no recompense. Not a surprise.

What this person failed to tell me in our meeting but what I already knew is that my estrogen levels were really high, and my progesterone and testosterone needed increasing. She failed to tell me that I was insulin resistant and that I should see a specialist for that, that my cortisol levels were doing a roller coaster ride on a daily basis causing Cyclical Cushing's Syndrome, and that this was potentially life threatening. She also failed to mention my high inflammation levels or my compromised antibodies. Oh, she did catch my low Vitamin D levels though.

I should have bolted for the door when the receptionist asked me to prepay.
I had another chance to leave when the nurse came to get me and she was at least 20 years older than the picture on her new website...

In moments of desperation you will hold onto the belief that these people will help you...Until they don't. I held on.

I knew I'd been had almost immediately. Cripes ... $775 can get me laser eye surgery or an all inclusive week in Mexico.

It is of course hard to not trust someone that paints such a great picture of what they do for all the world to see...Heed my warning. Get testimonials from previous clients, do research and trust your instinct. Think long and hard before you even pay a $200 deposit to these people, because it's usually non refundable.

In good news, I returned to my previous clinic to see my original Dr. and he got me back on track, where I'm now making good headway. Of course there will always be bumps in the road, but now you will be be aware. If it seems far too good to be true, and it costs you a month's mortgage payment, it is too good to be true; run (okay, stroll steadily) for the hills.

In Summation

If you have made it this far, then you have absolutely got the resolve to thrive, and not just survive.

Remember, nothing will change overnight. You must be absolutely invested in your own well being and any outcomes that you strive to work toward. Roll with any setbacks and chalk them down to experience, but never dwell on something that didn't work for you, because there is always an alternative.

Add an exercise regimen, adjust your diet, add new medication, visit your Dr....fire your Dr. nap, adjust your medication, get a new Dr. travel, paint, read...Not all at once, obviously, but you know what to do.

Slow and steady really can win this race.

I believe in you...and so should you.

GOOD LUCK

Recipes

Comforting Chili

1 lb of ground beef (can be switched for turkey or chicken)
3-4 jalapeno peppers, with seeds finely sliced
1 handful of fresh chopped cilantro or parsley
20 cherry tomatoes cut in half
1 can tomato paste/ tube of tomato puree
I-2 cups of water
2 sachets of beef bouillon or 2 beef oxo cubes
Dried chili seeds to taste
A dash of tabasco sauce as required
Pink himalayan salt and ground black pepper to taste

Enough rice to make 6 small servings
Bring a pan of water to the boil Add a generous knob of butter and the rice Turn the heat to a simmer and cook with the lid on until ready You may need to add more water Stir regularly

Place to one side and cool

Brown the ground beef in a small amount of water
Add the jalapeno and the tomatoes and cook at a
medium heat for 10 minutes Gently add everything
else and simmer for up to 2 hours with the lid on,
stirring and adding water as required.

Allow to cool, combine with rice and package in pre
marked bags or containers

For delicious vegetarian or vegan alternatives you
can use tofu, extra vegetables (carrots and
cauliflower work well with all of these recipes) and
vegetable stock, instead of beef bouillon

Quick and Easy Cottage Pie

For Shepherds Pie, you just switch ground beef out for ground lamb.

1 lb ground beef.
1 large can chopped tomatoes with no additives or 6-8 fresh beef tomatoes, cut each one into eight pieces
1 small can tomato paste/ tube tomato puree
1 generous handful of fresh chopped parsley or two generous teaspoons of dried parsley
2 sachets beef bouillon or two beef oxo stock cubes
1 cup water
4 large carrots, washed/ or peeled cut into 1cm cubes
1 small swede/rutabaga peeled cut into 1 cm small cubes

4 baking potatoes, scrubbed or peeled. Cut into 1 inch cubes.

Pinch of freshly ground black pepper and pinch of pink himalayan salt

Cover prepared potatoes with water in a saucepan and cook until soft.
Drain and mash with a dash of cream (35%) a generous knob of butter, and a pinch of salt.. Place to one side.

Brown the ground beef in a deep, oven proof skillet, with a little of the water.

Add carrots and swede/rutabaga and a little more water. Cook for 15 minutes with the lid on the pan, at a simmer, stir occasionally.
Add all other ingredients and stir together well.
Do not make the mixture too runny. Only add more water if it appears stodgy.
Cook for a further 5-10 minutes.

Remove from the heat and make sure the mix is level in the pan, then spread the mashed potatoes evenly on top of the mixture, place carefully in the oven on a centre shelf and cook at 410f for 25 minutes.

Cool, and place food in 6 separate portions ready to freeze.

You can use ziplock bags, small plastic ziplock reusable containers or the store brand equivalent for freshness.

Use a sharpie to write the date and contents on the packaging, before you put the food in.

Swift Spaghetti Sauce

1 lb ground beef, turkey or chicken
2 large cloves or 4 med cloves of garlic, peeled and
crushed   Wild is preferable
1 can tomato paste/ tube tomato puree
1 large can of chopped tomatoes, no additives or 6-8
ripe beef tomatoes cut into 8 pieces
1 cup of water
2 teaspoons of mixed dried herbs or a generous
bunch of fresh chopped basil and parsley
6 medium-large mushrooms peeled and sliced
2 sachets beef bouillon or two beef oxo cubes
Ground black pepper and himalayan pink salt to
taste
Dash or two of Worcestershire Sauce if preferred

Spaghetti can be prepared on the same day and
added to the freezer mix, or fresh on the day of
consuming You'll need enough for 6 med sized
portions if you are adding to the freezable food

Bring a pan of water to the boil, add a dash of salt
and place spaghetti into the water
Cook until tender Drain and serve
If you are adding to the freezer food, you may find it
easier to chop it a little

Gently brown the ground beef in a little of the water.
Add the crushed garlic and chopped mushrooms
after just a few minutes. Cook for 5-8 minutes on
medium and then gently stir in the remaining
ingredients Add water as necessary
Simmer for 15-20 minutes on a medium to low heat

Cool and split into 6 portions
Place in freezer bags, or reusable freezable
containers that are pre-marked with the date and
contents

Useful Contacts

For those looking for further and more in-depth information

www.nationalmssociety.org Multiple Sclerosis

www.arthritis.org Arthritis and FMS

www.stopthethyroidmadness.com Thyroid, Adrenal, Autoimmune and Endocrine

www.hypothyroidmom.com Thyroid, Adrenal, Autoimmune and Endocrine

www.thyroidnation.com Thyroid, Adrenal, Autoimmune and Endocrine

www.lupus.org Autoimmune

www.ccfa.org Digestive and Autoimmune

www.pcos.org Endocrine and Autoimmune

www.parkinson.org Parkinsons Disease

www.cancer.org Cancer

www.mentalhealth.org Depression and Mental Health

www.diabetes.org Diabetes and Endocrine

www.aad.org Skin

www.heartandstroke.org Circulatory and Heart

https://cts.lung.ca/ Circulatory and Breathing

Most of the links provided will lead you to the North American sites.
Each of these websites provide invaluable links to similar or connected illnesses, and to chapters of their organizations in your region or Country.

For Bio Identical Hormone Replacement Therapy research your local practitioners.

NOTE: $300 is the standard charge for an initial consultation. Persons charging much more than this should not be contacted.

DO NOT always trust the testimonials on private clinic websites.

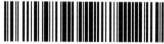
64209403R00087

Made in the USA
Charleston, SC
23 November 2016